Dream Interpretation as a Psychotherapeutic Technique

Frederick L. Coolidge PhD
Professor of Psychology
University of Colorado at Colorado Springs

Foreword by
Ernest Hartmann MD

Radcliffe Publishing
Oxford • Seattle

Radcliffe Publishing Ltd
18 Marcham Road
Abingdon
Oxon OX14 1AA
United Kingdom

www.radcliffe-oxford.com
Electronic catalogue and worldwide online ordering facility.

British Library Cataloguing in Publication Data

A catalogue record for this book is available from the British Library.

ISBN-10 1 84619 017 7
ISBN-13 978 1 84619 017 9

Typeset by Ann Buchan (Typesetters), Middlesex
Printed and bound by T J International Ltd, Padstow, Cornwall

Contents

Foreword

Dr Coolidge has written an excellent and very accessible book on dream interpretation and the use of dreams in psychotherapy.

The book succinctly summarizes the history of dream interpretation from the Ancients, through Freud and Jung, to the present. The author does not insist on a new interpretation technique of his own, but makes helpful comments on each technique, and then suggests a synthesis of various modes of interpretation, offering useful, flexible guidelines for an approach to dreams.

The book is written clearly, in textbook style, with summaries of the main points at the end of each chapter. There are many examples of the author's approach to individual dreams.

I would recommend this book to any student or beginning therapist interested in working with dreams.

Ernest Hartmann MD
Professor of Psychiatry
Tufts University
Author of *Dreams and Nightmares* (Perseus, 2001)
March 2006

About the author

According to psychologist Alfred Adler, our lives are often framed around our earliest memories. My earliest memory was a nightmare. At about the age of two, I dreamt that my aunt, my father, and I were driving in my father's Ford and trying to go around the rear entrance of a hospital where my brother had just been born. In my dream, my aunt sat with me in the back seat. We drove by a jumble of trash cans, parked the car, and then walked down a long corridor. We sat on a hard bench waiting for my mother and new brother. While in college, a psychology professor asked us to recall our earliest memory, and I recalled that dream. I called my mother shortly after and asked her about my recollection. Indeed, she said, my father drove around the back of the hospital where the garbage was placed. My aunt did accompany my father, and we did wait in a long corridor lined with benches.

As an undergraduate at the University of Florida, I worked in a NASA-sponsored sleep laboratory for three years. I then built and ran my own sleep laboratory for four years while in Florida's Psychology PhD program. My masters' thesis determined the feasibility of learning a foreign language during sleep (which I published in the *Australian Journal of Psychology* in 1972). My doctoral dissertation examined the relationship between various sleep stages and verbal and nonverbal memory (which I presented as a paper to the American Psychological Association convention in 1979).

I am now a Professor of Psychology at the University of Colorado at Colorado Springs. A while ago, one of my students (whose father was an oncologist) brought me the dreams of 14 dying cancer patients, up to one month before their death. She and I analyzed these dreams, and we published the study in *Omega: The Journal of Death and Dying* in 1983. A short time later, another student told me he had the recurring dream that his teeth were falling out. We examined the literature and found the dream to be at least 2000 years old. We then examined the personality characteristics of other college students with that same dream and published that study in *Psychological Reports* in 1984. Recently, I completed a paper reviewing the consequences for cognition of ground sleep in early hominids (about two million years ago).

I have also been trained as a Clinical Psychologist, and I worked as a Forensic Psychologist for the State of Florida. Through all of these experiences, I am able to present the interpretation of dreams from a broad scientific yet clinical perspective. In 1999, I presented a workshop at the American Psychological

Association annual convention entitled, 'Dream Interpretation as a Psychotherapeutic Technique.' Thus, I find that my fascination with sleep and dreams continues.

F.L.C.

Book Cover: The symbols on the cover are the consonantal sounds for the Egyptian hieroglyphic 'upshw' which means to sleep or dream (Budge, 1978). The topmost symbol is the feather of an ostrich (for a 'shw' sound). Below it are the horns of an ox ('wp' sound). Below it is a sitting stool of reed matting ('p' sound), and a set of crossed sticks. The latter is a determinative that tells the reader that the word is an action.

To the memory of my father, Paul Lawrence Coolidge
and to my mother, Dolores J Coolidge

CHAPTER I

An introduction to dream interpretation

The purpose of this book is to help you interpret dreams. While the self-analysis of dreams is possible and can be beneficial, the interpretation of a person's dreams by a trained therapist probably has greater benefits. This book, therefore, is designed both for therapists who wish to use dream analysis as a psychotherapeutic technique and for laypeople who are interested in the field of dream interpretation. The ability to understand dreams is certainly not restricted to therapists. Anyone, properly motivated, can gain insights and benefit from exploring the meaning of dreams. There have been many dream interpretation books, the first of them (that we have knowledge of) dating as far back as 4000 to 5000 years ago. It will be the underlying philosophy of this book to provide the reader with a solid scientific foundation for the interpretation of dreams. Also, this book will provide guidelines for ethical psychotherapeutic interpretation of dreams. Although it has already been stated that anyone could benefit from dream self-analysis, it seems reasonable to assume that one could benefit more from dream analysis with a trained professional. If it is true that some dreams symbolize deeper meanings, issues, and conflicts, then the same processes (defenses) that change these issues into dream images may prevent us from becoming aware of them while we are awake. A therapist who uses dream interpretation techniques may help people face difficult issues, ones that we might avoid on our own, or even ones of which we may not be consciously aware.

This book may be conceived of as having four sections. After the introduction, the first section provides a physiological foundation for the scientific nature of sleep and dreams. The second section provides a historical, cultural, and religious background for dream interpretation. As noted earlier, there are dream interpretation books dating back approximately 4500 years or more. Some of the earliest written records, of any kind, contain reports of dreams. Dreams have also played a fascinating history in many major religions including Judaism, Christianity, Hinduism, Buddhism, Islam, Mormonism, and others. History is also replete with reports that God speaks through dreams, and this topic is discussed in greater detail. The third major section of this book covers more modern and highly influential dream theorists. An overview is provided of the dream theories of Sigmund Freud, Carl Jung, and Fritz Perls. A summary of their dream interpretation techniques is also provided at the ends of those three chapters. Finally, the fourth section provides a synthesis of dream interpretation techniques that can be applied in psychotherapy and daily life. Numerous examples are also given.

Myths of dream interpretation: a dream glossary

Throughout this book, the scientific and ethical interpretation of dreams will be stressed. So what constitutes a myth with regard to dream interpretation? To begin, there is very little or no scientific evidence that dreams may be interpreted by a universal glossary. In other words, you cannot look up a dream image (like a lobster) in a book and find out that it means that you will soon experience difficulties in your life. There is a plethora of books that contain glossaries but none are based on any scientific evidence. Dream book glossaries may be entertaining, and interestingly they have ancient historical roots (probably dating back at least to 2500 B.C.) but this approach is highly unscientific. *See* Figure 1.1 for a 1931 dream glossary book.

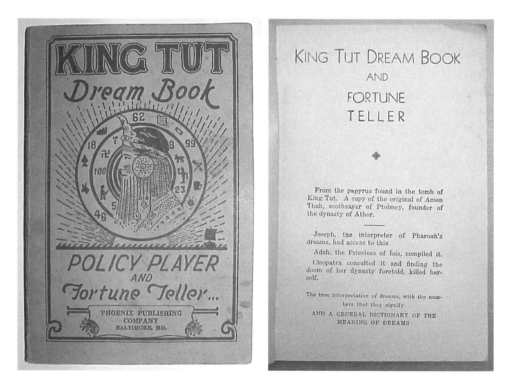

Figure 1.1: King Tut Dream Book

Self-dream analysis at the least might also be deemed inefficient, as hinted at earlier, it is a central idea in this book that trained dream interpretation therapists are probably more efficient at getting at important psychological issues than we would obtain by interpreting dreams on our own. Experienced dream interpreters with proper training may be able to see through unconscious defenses and make connections between events and issues that individuals on their own could not or would not see or make.

Psychology: the field of dreams

Psychology is probably one of the most appropriate fields to host studies of dream interpretation. Certainly other disciplines, like biology, chemistry, and evolutionary sciences contribute to the understanding of dreams, but psychology, since its inception, has been a home for the study of dreaming and dream interpretation. Wilhelm Wundt (1804–1899), a German psychologist, has often been credited with founding the scientific discipline of psychology in 1879. What did Wundt have to say about dreams? Wundt (1896) believed that dreaming was a kind of temporary insanity. Dreaming is a hallucination, he wrote. He believed dreaming gave the normal person a glimpse of what a mental disturbance would be like. He dismissed premonition dreams as baseless. And vivid dreams, Wundt thought, were most often caused by indigestion. As for the general physiological nature of sleep, Wundt thought it vital and originating from the central nervous system.

William James (1842–1910), an American psychologist, wrote *Principles of Psychology*, published in 1890. He is often credited with either co-establishing psychology along with Wundt or establishing psychology in America. In his epic textbook (James, 1890/1981) he had only one reference to dreams, and it is a mere footnote. Nevertheless, he was much more sympathetic to the psychological meaning of dreams than Wundt. James wrote that dreams might give us a glimpse of the 'spiritual world.' He noted that dreams throughout history have been considered divine revelations and often furnish us with mythologies and religious themes. Dreaming, he believed, was the other half of our 'larger universe.' The natural world consisted of our waking perceptions, and our supernatural world consisted of our dream images, and together they form our larger universe.

John B. Watson (1878–1935), another American psychologist is credited with being the founder of the behavioristic paradigm. One would not expect a behaviorist to be sympathetic to dreaming, but, surprisingly, Watson was. In his textbook, *Psychology from the Standpoint of a Behaviorist* (Watson, 1919), he stated that dream analysis often reveals emotional tensions. 'Dreams,' he wrote, 'are a part of a person's sum total of reactions. They are as good indicators of the nature of his personality, of his stresses and strains and emotional life generally, as are any of his other activities.'

A new theory on the origin and meaning of dreams: Ernest Hartmann

Ernest Hartmann is a contemporary sleep and dream researcher. One of his earliest works was *The Biology of Dreaming* (Hartmann, 1967), which I read while an undergraduate. He is a world-renowned expert on the biology of dreaming, but more recently in his career he extended his interests to dreams and nightmares. At the American Psychological Association convention in Boston in 1999, I was finally able to see him speak in public. He began with an introduction that produced an audible impression on the audience when he said he had met Sigmund Freud. Because Freud died in 1939 and Hartmann did not look old enough, I was immediately skeptical. He put all our skepticisms to rest when he said that his father carried him in his arms at the age of two to meet the famous Dr. Freud.

Hartmann's (1998) new theory of dreaming builds on many previous theories and is consistent with my own dream analysis principles. First, he affirms there is no glossary of meaning. He believes that dreaming connects different thoughts. In that regard, he believes it may not be completely different than waking consciousness in that we also make connections between different thoughts and ideas while we are awake. However, he thought that dreaming allows us to make more creative and broad connections than when awake. He thought that dreaming tends to avoid well worn, 'tightly woven or overlearned regions of the mind.' He believed that this process of connecting was not random, but that it was guided by the emotions and emotional concerns of the dreamer. He saw dreams as providing a context for emotions, and, in his own words, he said, 'dreaming *contextualizes* emotion.' Part of this contextualization, he believed, was the ability of dreaming to note subtle similarities and to create metaphors for our emotional states. Thus, dreams create a story based on our emotions and psychological issues. Finally, Hartmann believed that the contextualization process thus served a purpose. By integrating new material into our dreaming consciousness and our waking consciousness, dreaming may help us become aware of problems, may help us solve them, may help us to be creative, and may calm emotional storms.

In the summary of his talk, Hartmann impressed me with a final thought. 'With dreams begin responsibilities,' he said. He told us that he liked the vagueness and uncertainty of the statement. At the same time, he thought that its roots went way back into the sands of time. He questioned whether it was to be interpreted as referring to our dreams when we sleep, or whether it was to be applied to our daydreams and imaginings. He did note, however, that if one had a big, powerful dream, one could sit back and simply say, 'Wow, that was incredible!' or he said:

> You can stop smoking, you can create a new machine, a painting, a sonata, or a new religion.

You can change your life. You are free, I suppose, to do something or to do nothing at all. It is your dream. In dreams begin responsibilities.

Summary

1 There is no scientific evidence for a glossary approach to dream interpretation, e.g., if you dream of your teeth falling out, it means you will die.
2 Dream interpretation has a rich and ancient history.
3 Dream interpretation is probably more efficient and beneficial when conducted by a trained therapist and a client than by a self-analysis of dreams.
4 Dreams may provide a context for our emotions.
5 With dreams begin responsibilities.

CHAPTER 2

The biological and evolutionary foundations of sleep and dreams

Guide of mortal man to wisdom,
he who has ordained the law,
knowledge won through suffering.
Drop, drop – in our sleep, upon the heart sorrow falls, memory's pain,
and to us, though against our very will, even in our despite,
comes wisdom
by the awful grace of God.
Aeschylus, 454 B.C., in the play *Agamemnon*

Please don't spoil my day, I'm miles away, and after all I'm only sleeping.
The Beatles (Lennon & McCartney, 1966)

Discovery of REM sleep

It is interesting to think that about 50 years ago the scientific study of sleep and dreams received a tremendous boost. Despite written records of dreams that date back over 4500 years, it was not until 1953 that University of Chicago sleep researchers Kleitman and his doctoral student Aserinsky discovered that their human sleep subjects not only slowly moved their eyes while falling asleep but also began to move their eyes rapidly during sleep. Aserinsky first noticed these eyes movements in sleeping infants. Later, in their studies with adults, they found these eye movements (called *REM* for *rapid eye movements*) coincided with the most vivid dreams throughout the entire sleep period. Aserinsky and Kleitman used an electroencephalograph (EEG) in order to measure their subjects' sleep. The EEG is a sophisticated machine used to amplify the tiny amounts of electrical activity produced primarily by the surface of the brain, the cortex. Now, sleep researchers regularly attach electrodes not only about their subjects' heads but also they place two electrodes about the outer area of each eye socket in order to measure the presence of REM sleep. Quickly after Aserinsky and

Kleitman's important discovery, the hypothesis became popular that a human's sleep could be divided into five sleep stages, four of them containing *non-REM sleep* and one containing REM sleep (e.g., Dement, 1972). Animal researchers also looked for the presence of REM sleep, and they found that almost all mammals have REM sleep, and nearly all reptiles, fishes, and birds do not.

One might wonder, as the ancients actually did, what animals might dream about. In fact, Freud in his most influential work, *Die Traumdeutung (The Interpretation of Dreams)*, wrote that he himself did not know what animals dreamed of but a student had made him aware of a proverb that asked what do geese dream of, and the reply was 'corn,' 'pigs of acorns,' and 'hens of millet.' To be as scientifically correct as currently possible, it should be noted that it appears that thoughts, thinking, thought fragments, and perhaps even brief dreams, may occur throughout the sleep period, particularly across non-REM sleep. So, when I stated earlier that REM sleep occurs mostly in mammals, this does not mean that reptiles, fishes, and birds do not dream. However, the popular conception, even among scientists, is that when we speak of dreaming, we are referring to the vivid thoughts and emotions that accompany REM sleep.

And, furthermore, we might wonder how scientists could even hope to approach this problem of what animals dream about, because we know that animals cannot exactly tell us, at least in our language. There have been, however, a few ingenious research attempts to answer this question. Jouvet (1999), a French sleep researcher from the University of Lyon, cut the descending neural pathways that are responsible for the inhibition of motor movements during REM sleep in cats. He then observed that during REM sleep these cats appeared to act out the stalking of their prey and would even jump upon their imaginary dinner, kill it, and eat it. Other researchers have trained monkeys to press a lever while awake to specific visual stimuli. Later during sleep, the monkeys again pressed the lever, and it can be tenuously assumed that the monkeys were responding to the same but now internalized visual stimuli in their dreams. Wilson, of MIT, and McNaughton, of the University of Arizona, put electrodes into the hippocampus of rats (Wilson and McNaughton, 1994). The hippocampus is a seahorse-shaped structure lying underneath the surface of the cortex on both sides of the brain (bilateral), and, in rats at least, it is thought to be responsible for spatial memory. They then taught the rats to successfully run a maze and observed particular patterns of neuronal firing in response to certain parts of running the maze. Later while the rats were in non-REM sleep, the hippocampal neurons again displayed the previous response firing patterns. These findings suggest that rats' brains are active during sleep, even non-REM sleep, and yes, laboratory rats may 'dream' of mazes.

Stages of sleep

After Aserinsky and Kleitman's discovery of a distinct stage of sleep for vivid

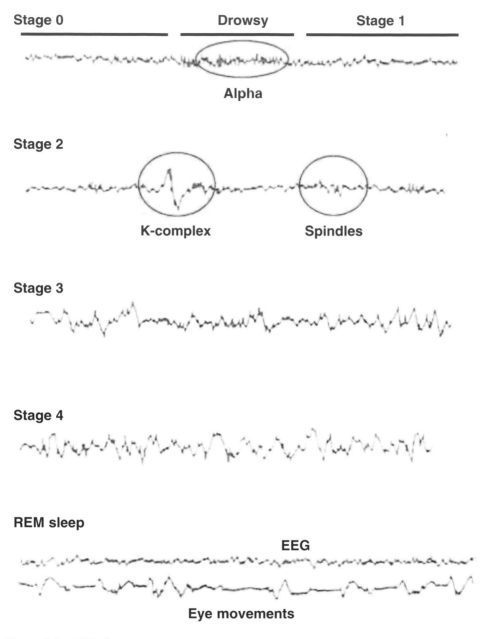

Figure 2.1: EEG sleep stages

dreaming, sleep researchers settled down to the present thinking that sleep consists of five different stages. They are as follows (*see* Figure 2.1 for examples of
the EEG sleep stages).

Stage 0

In this stage we are still awake but resting with our eyes closed. On the EEG will appear a very beautiful semi-symmetrical wave, known as *alpha*. It was first described in 1929 by Berger, a German psychiatrist. Alpha waves are of moderately large amplitude, and occur in most people at a frequency of about 10 Hz (cycles per second) with a range from 9 to 12 Hz. Alpha waves are all fairly similar and rhythmic which adds to their beauty. Alpha is most clearly produced over the back part (posterior) of the skull (over the occipital lobes or the primary visual processing part of the cortex). Most people produce alpha but approximately 30% do not, and we do not know the reasons why. I still remember my disappointment when I was first working in a sleep lab and wired myself up, plugged myself into the EEG, and found that I did not produce alpha.

When sleep subjects are producing alpha, and they either open their eyes, or they are asked to think about a complex thought like figuring out the square root of 26 in their head, alpha is either diminished or eliminated. This phenomenon is known as alpha blocking. Because alpha is typically produced when subjects are awake but resting, it has become popularly associated with being synonymous with a state of relaxation. However, there is little scientific evidence to support this speculation. It has even been argued that alpha is not a brain wave but an artifact of the eye muscle potential between the two eyes. In all of our sleep experiments at the University of Florida, we first conducted a brief screening of all human volunteers, and eliminated those who did not produce alpha waves, or, as we said, were not alpha dominant. Thus, during any of our sleep experiments, we could tell almost to the second when a subject had awakened, by the presence of alpha. Actually, most of our subjects did awaken periodically during the night. However, these brief periods of alpha lasted only seconds, perhaps, when a subject might change positions in bed, or roll over, and they rarely if ever remembered that they had awakened.

Interestingly, most subjects do not sleep well their first night in a sleep lab. After all, they are in a strange place, with a strange bed and pillow, have their head full of electrodes that have been pasted on, and each electrode is connected by long wires bundled together, the sleep subjects are plugged into a panel at the head of the bed, and finally, they are told to relax and go to sleep! Thus, the first night's data from many sleep subjects is tossed out, or the EEG machine will not even be turned on, because the subject's first night will be highly atypical of their regular sleep, with many more awakenings than usual, less deep sleep, and less REM sleep. This phenomenon is known as the *first night effect*, and we have all probably experienced it when we spend our first night away from home on a vacation, business or camping trip. We typically wake up in the morning and complain that we did not sleep well or that we were up all night. The first night effect may occur even when we may feel relaxed in a nice hotel. As Seuss noted in Geisel (1962):

What a fine night for sleeping! From all that I hear,
It's the best night for sleeping in many a year.
They're even asleep in the Zwieback Motel!
And people don't usually sleep there too well.
The beds are like rocks and, as everyone knows,
The sheets are too short. They won't cover your toes.
SO, if people are actually sleeping in THERE...
It's a great night for sleeping! It must be the air.
Dr. Seuss's Sleep Book (Geisel, 1962)

This little poem probably inadvertently notes the association between restless sleep and a motel. Although the author blames the beds and sheets, the blame more than likely goes to the first night effect. Humans, however, adapt quickly to a new environment, and the second night of sleep is much more often typical of our regular sleep patterns.

There is a second waking brain wave called the *beta rhythm* (13 to 30 Hz), which was also first described by Berger (1930). Beta consists of low voltage waves, rapidly occurring, and appearing irregular. When people are awake, they typically alternate between alpha and beta, and beta occurs all over the scalp, even over the occipital lobes when alpha is blocked. It is believed that alpha and beta waves (and all other EEG waves) are created by large clusters of brain cells in the cerebral cortex (the upper layers of the brain) as a result of postsynaptic activity. It is also thought that the voltage of a wave will increase if the synaptic activity of the cells is synchronized. Thus, alpha is believed to be the result of synchronized neuronal activity while beta is the product of desynchronized activity.

A third waking brain wave is called *theta* (4 to 7 Hz). Theta can also serve as a transition wave between sleep and wakefulness. It is observed while people are awake but also as people get drowsy, their attention begins to drift, or sometimes when they engage in creative thinking.

Stage 1

This is usually the first and the lightest (easiest from which to awaken) of the sleep stages. It accounts for about 10% of the total normal sleep period. Stage 1 usually consists of brain waves that are of low voltage, irregular, and desynchronized, with some brief periods of theta activity. Theta activity more often occurs while we are awake so this is one of the reasons stage 1 is considered a transition stage from wakefulness to sleep.

One of the more debatable experiences during sleep may occur before or during stage 1 sleep, and that is the *hypnagogic state*. This few-minutes-long period is well known, however, and occurs when we start to experience the transition from wakefulness to sleep. Usually people report a floating sensation accompanied by a slow loosening of thoughts and weird or bizarre imagery. It is debatable because the EEG correlates of these weird thought fragmentations are not well established nor have the subject's reports been analyzed along with EEG monitoring.

Interestingly, the onset of sleep in nearly all primates is often accompanied by the *hypnic* or *hypnagogic jerk*, which is a sudden muscle reflexive movement that frequently awakens the sleeper. Although the ultimate cause of the hypnic jerk is unknown, a common hypothesis is that it is an archaic reflex to the brain's misinterpreting the muscle relaxation accompanying the onset of sleep as a signal that the sleeping primate is falling out of a tree. The reflex may also have had selective value by having the sleeper readjust or review his or her sleeping position in a nest or on a branch in order to assure that a fall did not occur.

Stage 2

The EEG changes from stage 1 to stage 2 are subtle. However, stage 2 is fairly easy to identify because of the distinctive presence of *sleep spindles* (13 to 16 Hz). They are of moderate voltage so they stand out against the general low voltage background of stage 2, and they appear in bursts of about one to two seconds in length. Spindles occur about once or twice every minute. Stage 2 is the most prevalent stage of sleep and accounts for about 50% of our total sleep. It is also evenly distributed throughout the sleep period. Stage 2 can also be considered a transition stage from and to any of the other stages of sleep, such as from lighter sleep to deeper sleep to REM sleep.

Because stage 2 is so prevalent and evenly distributed throughout a sleep period, my masters' thesis Chair C. M. Levy and I chose it to present common Russian words paired with their English equivalents to English-only college students to see if they could learn during sleep (Levy, Coolidge, and Stabb, 1972). We found that the students could recognize the correct answers when awakened in the morning significantly better than chance. However, the actual amount of learning beyond chance was so minimal and it took so many repeated trials to learn that we concluded that *sleep learning* was not worth the effort.

Stage 2 also has a second distinctive brain wave known as a *K-complex* which usually consists of a single large voltage burst beginning with a negative deflection followed by a smaller positive one. K-complexes do occur during wakefulness but usually only in response to some external stimuli. Their purpose during stage 2 sleep is unknown.

Stage 3

This stage is at least partially artifactual. When I was learning to score EEG sleep stages, I always did poorly on identifying it. So, rather than frustrating myself with the official definition for its identification, I began to go directly to identifying stage 4 (which is very easy to find) and then I would back up exactly two minutes before the onset of stage 4 and call it stage 3. Immediately my correct identification scores soared above 90%.

Less cynically, stage 3 officially contains some stage 2 activity like spindles and K-complexes, and we start to see the first appearance of some stage 4 activity, *delta waves* (.5 to 3 Hz). Delta waves are high amplitude waves, the highest of all the sleep stages. They are also very slow, only one to three peaks in one second (contrast this to a spindle with up to 16 peaks a second). Thus, delta wave sleep is also called *slow-wave sleep*.

Stage 4

Delta wave activity dominates this stage (greater than 50% of a one-minute period). Stage 3 and stage 4 together account for about 15% of our total sleep. A large majority of stage 4 occurs during the first third of the night. Stage 4 is also considered the deepest stage of sleep because sleepers are the most difficult to awaken from this stage. If they are asked if they are dreaming vividly, they almost always say no. If they are asked if they are thinking about something, they more often say no but sometimes say yes. The thoughts they report, however, are usually brief and fragmentary. The latter is also true of stage 2 and 3 as well. The subjects rarely, if ever, report vivid dreaming but do report some thinking or fragmentary thoughts.

During stage 4 the parasympathetic system (which is part of the autonomic nervous system and controls vegetative functions like digestion) predominates, and the gastrointestinal system becomes more active. The cardiovascular system slows, including decreases in heart rate, blood pressure, and respiration.

Interestingly, stage 3 and stage 4 decrease across the lifespan. Up to 25% of 50-year-olds have no stage 4 sleep whatsoever, and this percentage increases with increasing age. Also, as we age, the number of sleep awakenings increases dramatically, there is an increase in the lighter stages of sleep, and naps tend to increase.

REM sleep

It is a somewhat contentious issue among sleep researchers as to whether REM sleep is associated with our most vivid dreams. Some would argue that dream stories can occur in other stages of sleep. I would agree. However, after my seven years of EEG, sleep, and dream research, I fall easily on the side of the argument that our most vivid dreams far more often occur in REM sleep, and thus, I take the position that dream sleep and REM sleep are almost, but not quite, synonymous. Another issue among sleep researchers is how long after falling asleep the first REM period occurs. Somewhere after the first hour of sleep and mostly before the second hour, the EEG appears to reflect stage 1 sleep. However, this event is actually the onset of REM sleep because the dormant EEG eye channels (recording muscle movements of the eyes) begin to show activity. There are also sudden changes in respiration, and blood pressure fluctuates wildly, as does heart rate.

Males get penile erections (and more often than not, the erections are not accompanied by erotic dreams). Similar to males, females have clitoral responses in REM sleep. In fact, when men complain of impotence (failure to get an erection when they wish to), a test to determine whether the impotence has an organic (clear physiological cause) or psychogenic (psychological cause) basis consists of simply determining whether the man gets an erection during REM sleep. If he does, then the cause of the impotence is thought to be psychogenic.

REM sleep accounts for about 25% of our total sleep. Infants spend about 50% of their total sleep in REM while the percentage drops to about 25% by the age of 6 to 10 years old and remains fairly stable throughout the rest of the lifespan. The first REM period is short, usually a few minutes in length, while subsequent REM periods increase in length to the point where the latter periods may last 20 minutes or more. A strong majority of REM sleep is obtained over the last third of the sleep period.

It borders on religious dogma to state that REM comes in 90 minute cycles, that is, every 90 minutes beginning from the onset of sleep, we have a REM period. In my years of sleep lab research and experience, I have found that there is tremendous variation in REM cyclicity. One time, I noted to a graduate student colleague that the sleeping subject we were EEG monitoring had his first REM onset after about two and a half to three hours. Without hesitation, my colleague explained that this subject had 'skipped' his first REM period, and the first REM period we just observed was really his second. What seems universally clear is that most of our REM sleep occurs over the last third of the night, and I think the classic '90-minute REM cycle' has such great variation that it becomes difficult for me to use it even as a rough rule-of-thumb.

Another interesting characteristic of the REM sleep occurs at its onset. *Muscle atonia* (loss of muscle tone or muscle 'paralysis') is a physiological response that occurs with the onset of REM sleep. Jouvet (1980) explored the role of inhibitory neurons upon voluntary muscle systems in preventing these systems from acting out dreams. Morrison (1983) demonstrated that selective destruction of these inhibitory neurons allowed cats to act out predatory actions, presumably the content of their REM dreams. Some sleeping people can become aware of this muscle paralysis during REM sleep, and their accompanying dream themes often reflect the interpretation of muscle atonia, such as being paralyzed by aliens or being crushed by ghosts (e.g., Wing, Lee, and Chen, 1994). In their study of over 600 Chinese undergraduates, over 93% had heard of the ghost oppression dream and 37% claimed to have experienced it.

It has also been suggested that one of the most common themes of all adult dreams, falling, may in part occur because of the sleeper's interpretation of the complete muscle atonia that accompanies the onset of REM sleep (e.g., Van de Castle, 1994). The other suspicion, of course, is that the falling theme is connected to our arboreal hominid origins, as falling out of a tree was an event that an early hominid should not have taken lightly nor have easily forgotten (e.g., Sagan, 1977).

For some sleep researchers, REM sleep appears to be a very different experience than non-REM sleep, not only physiologically, but, as I have already stated, psychologically as well. For example, the dreams during REM sleep are reported as far more vivid and real than dreams from other stages, and dreams from REM are reliably reported more than from any other stage of sleep. Some modern sleep researchers have even called it a third state of consciousness: they postulate wakefulness, sleep, and REM sleep. This trinity is actually an ancient one: early Hindu writings depicted vaiswanara (wakefulness), prajna (dreamless sleep), and taijasa (dream sleep).

Evolutionary history of sleep

Now that we have reviewed the established physiological definitions for sleep and dreams in both humans and animals, let us go back to an even more preliminary question: why do we sleep and how did sleep develop? On its surface, it does not appear that sleep would be a clear evolutionary advantage. Sleeping organisms are unaware or minimally aware of their external environment, they cannot reproduce, they cannot feed, and they move very little, thus making excellent prey. However, given the near universality of sleep in organisms, particularly as organisms become more complex, there must be some evolutionary advantage of sleep and of a sleep–wake cycle.

It is thought that non-REM sleep has existed for about 200 million years with the evolution of the first warm-blooded mammals. Dream sleep may have been in existence for about 150 million years, and probably made its first appearance along with mammals that started reproducing their young directly from the womb and not through the external hatching of eggs. At one point in graduate school, one of my doctoral professors, Wilse Webb, proposed that sleep, at least eight hours of it, was unnecessary. In a pilot study, we allowed human volunteers to sleep only two hours a night. However, they were so grouchy and ornery after two days, we terminated the study. Webb growled with disappointment but then brightened as he reasoned that sleep had evolved over millions and millions of years, and it was not a fair test of his theory to expect the need for sleep to go away in just two nights. Later, in 1975, Webb proposed that sleep and its concomitant lack of motor activity must have evolutionary adaptive value by protecting most sleeping organisms during darkness from predators they could not see and from cliffs and bogs hidden in the night. Thus, Webb argues that nonbehavior or not responding during darkness may be evolutionarily adaptive, and the evolution of sleep insures these periods of non-activity or 'rest.' Clearly some organisms, like night predators, or dusk and dawn feeders, have adjusted their own sleep–wake cycle uniquely in order to take maximum advantage of the availability of their food supply. Also, I might add that the metabolic costs of running and feeding an organism 24 hours a day, particularly across darkened periods, might not only be exorbitant but also less likely to lead to evolution than for organisms that incorporated rest cycles.

Webb further proposed that the deep, heavy stages of non-REM sleep served to knock us out to begin our non-responding period, and he believed that REM sleep evolved to wake us up. After all, he reasoned, the deepest stages of non-REM sleep occur in the first third of our sleep period and are the least likely to contain vivid dreams, while REM mostly occurs over the last third of our sleep period and contains our most vivid dreams. And just like a biological alarm clock, REM sleep is also accompanied by rapid changes in blood pressure, heart rate, respiration, penile erections in men, and clitoral parallels in women.

A more modern speculation for the differentiation of slow-wave and REM sleep comes from the work of Kavanau (2002). He proposed that as ambient temperatures during twilight portions of primitive sleep rose above an animal's core temperature, the thermoregulatory need for muscle contractions became superfluous. With the absence of muscle tone (muscle atony), he proposed that selection may have favored fast waves during nocturnal twilight sleep. These fast waves may have reinforced motor circuits of evolving warm-blooded organisms without the concomitant, sleep-disturbing muscle contractions. Through these and other mechanisms, twilight sleep may have become REM sleep, and the daylight sleep may have become slow-wave sleep and non-REM sleep.

The effects of the tree-to-ground sleep transition in the evolution of sleep stages and cognition

Because it appears to be reasonable to assume that non-responding periods in a 24-hour day–night cycle may be evolutionarily adaptive, it might even be additionally adaptive if the non-responding organism's brain was able to use these periods in some less intense yet still active fashion. With the help of a colleague, archaeologist Thomas Wynn (Coolidge and Wynn, in press), we have recently reviewed evidence from the evolutionary record that this indeed may be the case.

One of our most famous ancestors, Lucy (*Australopithecus afarensis*) who lived approximately 3 to 4 million years ago, has not even been assigned to our same genus, i.e., *Homo*. Indeed, at barely 3 feet tall and 60 pounds, she and her relatives probably slept in trees. This speculation is based in part on modern evidence of nest building in great apes such as chimpanzees, bonobos (pygmy chimps), and orang-utans. Sabater Pi, Veá, and Serrallonga (1997) proposed that early hominids such as Lucy had the perfect ancient hominid anatomy for sleeping in trees, that is, light weight and long slender limbs. Also, all modern great apes have slow-wave sleep and REM, and the latter varies from about 7% to 15% of their total sleep (Allison and Cicchetti, 1976). So we can only speculate that Lucy and her family slept at night, in trees, in nests, and had both slow-wave and REM sleep, although probably less of the latter than modern humans.

Early *Homo* and *Homo Erectus*

The earliest hominoid fossils assigned to our genus, *Homo*, indicate that its body was much like that of *Australopithecus afarensis*. It, too, then, retained features of a climbing anatomy, though it may have been more human-like than the australopithecines like Lucy. This speculation is in part based on the finding that early *Homo* had larger brains than australopithecines. The speculation is also based on the fact that at least one of the two *Homo* species, *Homo habilis,* made and used stone tools. *Homo habilis* means 'handyman.' However, it appears that the way the tools were made and used by *Homo habilis* can be duplicated by some modern apes (Wynn and McGrew, 1989). Thus, there is no overpowering reason to conclude that the earliest of *Homo* had given up sleeping in trees even though they had bigger brains than Lucy.

The next major evolutionary advance in the *Homo* line, *Homo erectus,* clearly did give up sleeping in trees. A 1.8 million-year-old African fossil of a boy, about 11 to 15 years old, shows that he was already about 5 feet 6 inches tall and probably weighed about 120 pounds, far too tall and heavy for sleeping in trees. His brain was also much larger than that of *Homo habilis*, and his stone tools were far more sophisticated. This dramatic change in appearance and in culture suggests that an important evolutionary leap had been made. Thomas Wynn and I suggest that the change from tree to ground sleep was no mere accoutrement. We propose that the sleep transition from tree to ground allowed increases in the deep, heavy slow-wave sleep of stages 3 and 4, and in REM sleep (Coolidge and Wynn, in press).

The latter changes, however, pose some interesting problems. As noted earlier, it is very difficult to awaken people from slow-wave sleep, and REM sleep is accompanied by muscle atonia (muscle paralysis). Thus, sleeping on the ground, while it may have released early human types to receive more delta and REM sleep, made them inordinately more susceptible to being preyed upon. In Chapter 4, I will present three major advantages that may have come from sleeping on the ground that far outweighed the increased danger.

Summary

1   Sleep scientists currently divide wakefulness and sleep on the basis of EEG activity primarily from the surface of the cortex.

2   Wakefulness is partially defined by three waves, alpha (8–12 Hz), beta (13–30 Hz), and theta (4–7 Hz). Alpha is best recorded when subjects are resting, eyes closed, and not thinking about anything in particular.

3   Stage 1 sleep consists of low voltage, irregular, and desynchronized brain waves with some brief periods of theta activity. It is considered a light stage of sleep, and it occupies about 10% of a total sleep period.

4   Stage 2 is also considered a light stage of sleep, and bursts of sleep spindles (13–16Hz) and K-complexes (large negative deflections in EEG activity) are its definitive signs. Stage 2 takes up about 50% of a total sleep period, and it is fairly evenly spread across a sleep period.

5   Stage 3 is a transition stage between Stage 2 and Stage 4. It is generally considered the start of slow-wave sleep as delta waves (1–3 Hz) become evident during this stage.

6   Stage 4 is considered the deepest and heaviest stage of sleep, and it is defined by the presence of delta waves. Sleepers in stage 4 are very difficult to awaken and rarely report vivid dreams. Stage 3 and 4 account for about 15% of a total sleep period, and a majority of slow-wave sleep occurs in the first third of a sleep period. People over the age of 60 years old begin to have little or no delta wave sleep.

7   REM (rapid eye movement) sleep is nearly synonymous with vivid dream sleep, although dreams are reported in most other stages of sleep. REM accounts for about 25% of one's total sleep, and a majority occurs during the last third of a sleep period.

8   It is suspected that when ancient hominids stopped sleeping in trees and began sleeping on the ground, slow-wave sleep and REM sleep may have expanded, which may have aided the evolution of humans.

CHAPTER 3

A brief history of dream interpretation

The earliest history of dream interpretation has an interesting, repeating theme: communication between God and people through dreams, and dream-like revelations or visions. Some of the earliest recordings of this type of dream come from the area of the Middle East. The following review is not meant to be comprehensive nor all-encompassing. It is offered as a sampling of the rich and varied influences that dreams and dream interpretation have played in many religions and cultures over a long period of written history. Undoubtedly, dreams and dream interpretation must have played an important role in even more ancient cultures, perhaps even over hundreds of thousands of years, although this history is unavailable to us.

Mesopotamians

The Mesopotamian people (from what is now Iraq) included the Sumerians who left some of the earliest pictographic writings dating back to about 3100 B.C. By 2700 B.C. they had developed a cuneiform type of writing, which consisted of indentations on clay cylinders and tablets. Among their stories of religion, business, and war are accounts of gods speaking through dreams. The Sumerian king Gudea, who ruled in about 2220 B.C., had his dreams preserved on two clay tablets and these tablets contain the story of a puzzling dream that he had and his search with the help of a goddess for its meaning. This record is one of the earliest examples of the connection between gods and dreams, and further, it shows the early belief that gods not only talk to people through dreams but also guide people to religious acts of worship.

Around 2000 B.C., the mythic hero Gilgamesh is mentioned for the first time in Sumerian cuneiform writings, and the epic is expanded in later Assyrian (about 650 B.C.) writings. Gilgamesh fights, slays monsters, and searches for the secret of immortality, and all the while Gilgamesh is guided by his dreams. In fact, the twelve tablets reporting the Gilgamesh epic also offer the first known recurring dreams by the same dreamer, and the notion that dreams may foretell future misfortune. The idea that dreams may be interpreted through different techniques is also reported in the Gilgamesh story, along with the interesting idea that dreams may be incubated, thus increasing the probability that a god might give someone guidance. Apparently, the Mesopotamians were well practiced in the technique of *incubation* or dream seeking. The incubant, who was often a ruler, would go to a temple designed for the purpose of having guiding or prophetic dreams. There the incubant would perform special rituals and recite special prayers before going to sleep. In the morning, if the incubant was unsuccessful, the rituals and prayers might be altered until the dreamer was successful in receiving the gods' message through a dream. The Mesopotamians not only tried to figure out what a dream might mean but also used the dream to prevent or change a future misfortunate event from occurring.

Van de Castle, a contemporary dream theorist, reported an interesting Mesopotamian ritual:

> The Mesopotamians...told their dreams to a lump of clay... The dreamer would take the lump of clay and rub it over his entire body, saying, 'Lump! In your substance my substance has been fused, and in my substance your substance has been fused!' The dreamer then told the clay all the dreams and said to it, 'As I shall throw you into the water, you will crumble and disintegrate, and may the evil consequences of all the dreams seen be gone, be melted away, and be many miles removed from my body.' ... These rituals were particularly common when the dream was a nightmare or involved forbidden activities or sexual practices. The disturbing content of such dreams could not be mentioned to others and had to be dispelled magically to ward off possible evil consequences.
>
> (Van de Castle, 1994; p. 51)

Egyptians

The Egyptians are thought to have been influenced by the Mesopotamians (although there is some controversy about who influenced whom) in their dream beliefs, particularly in the idea that gods communicate through dreams. The Chester Beatty Papyrus, which dates to 1250 B.C., contains about 200 of these Egyptian dreams. The Egyptians believed that dreams were sent by the gods for a number of purposes: dreams helped foretell the future, dreams guided and advised people in their waking endeavors, and dreams offered suggestions for medical treatments against disease and for injury. Egyptians looked for *omina* or special signs. The omina could be mundane signs like birds in flight or they could come from dreams. For example, if a person dreamt that they splattered themselves with their own urine, then this omina portended: 'He will forget what he has said.' Egyptians used a wide variety of rituals, besides dreams, to contact their gods, including putting messages in the mouths of dead black cats, but dreams were considered a very potent method of communicating with the gods. Like the Mesopotamians, Egyptians went to special incubation temples and specially trained priests called 'Masters of the Secret Things (pa-hery-tep)' would offer their interpretations of the dreams. The Masters of the Secret Things would offer particular rituals and prayers for inducing dreams, and they helped in interpreting the symbolism in the dreams. For example, the dream of death was given the contradictory interpretation as being a portent of a long life.

An Egyptian pharaoh Thutmose IV erected a large stela between the paws of the Sphinx at Giza in about 1450 B.C. The stela was discovered in 1818 and inscribed was the story that Thutmose, before he became ruler of Egypt, had been out hunting and fell asleep in the shadow of the Sphinx. He had a dream that the Sphinx opened its lips and spoke to him and said:

'Behold me, O Thutmose, for I am the Sun-god, the ruler of all peoples. Harmachis is my name, and Ra, and Khepera, and Tem. I am thy father, and thou art my son, and through me shall all good come upon thee if thou wilt hearken to my words. The land of Egypt shall be thine, and the North Land, and the South Land. In prosperity and happiness shalt thou rule for many years... It is as thou seest, the sands of the desert are over me. Do that quickly which I command thee, O my son Thutmose.'
(Breasted, 1912; p. 327)

Thutmose awoke and, as commanded, he cleared the sand from the Sphinx, and erected the stela in honor of his dream. The rest of the story on the stela is damaged and undecipherable. However, as the Sun god had promised, Thutmose became ruler of Egypt, and apparently he was well loved and presided during a prosperous period.

There are also 21 Egyptian papyri, known as the oracular amuletic decrees, dating to about 1000 B.C. to approximately 700 B.C. They were small, wrapped up tightly, and were worn around the owner's neck as an amulet. Two-thirds of them were worn by female owners. The owners commissioned scribes to include the owner's name, and the most common of the papyri were appeals to gods for promises of immunity from diseases. Interestingly, though, there was frequent mention of dreams. These appeals took a common form, and that was to 'make every dream which [he or she] has seen good, and make every dream which someone else has seen for [him or her] good.'

The Egyptian tradition of recording dreams continued through the later Greek and Roman influences upon its culture. In a discovery of clay tablets in Saqqara, Egypt in the late 1960s and early 1970s, demotic (a cursive version of hieroglyphics) writings dating from about 180 B.C. to about 140 B.C. revealed that a priest named Hor had recorded battles, made appeals to the current Ptolemy VI, and noted his own dreams. In one of these tablets, Hor appeals to the gods Seth and Horus for a 'truthful' dream and a prediction for a beneficent future (Ray, 1976).

Jewish and Christian writings

In the Old Testament of the Bible, and in a story that may predate Thutmose' time, the first mention of a dream occurs in the book of Genesis. According to the Bible, Jacob, the son of Isaac and the grandson of Abraham, went on a journey to escape his brother Esau's death threat, and one night Jacob slept with a stone under his head. In Chapter 28:12–14, the following story is told:

> And he had a dream, and behold, a ladder was set on the earth with its top reaching to heaven; and behold, the angels of God were ascending and descending on it. And behold, the Lord stood above it and said, 'I am the Lord, the God of your father Abraham and the God of Isaac; the land on which you lie, I will give it to you and to your descendants. Your descendants shall also be like the dust of the earth, and you shall spread out to the west and to the east and to the north and to the south; and in you and in your descendants shall all the families of the earth be blessed.'

There are some fascinating similarities between these two tales. First, of course, is that God has communicated to a mortal through a dream. Second, God promises prosperity to both of the dreamers. Third, both stories curiously have God mentioning the direction of the dreamer's future rule (or its length and breadth, depending on the translation). Fourth, both dreamers are commanded by God to do some religious duty (in Genesis 35:1 Jacob is later commanded by God to build an altar where he had the dream). We might speculate that either God was consistent in using dreams as a mode of communication in about 2000 B.C. to 1500 B.C. or, at least, the dreams contain common archetypal themes: God's dream communication, the promises of prosperity, prediction of future events, and religious duty.

Later in the Book of Genesis, Jacob's son Joseph becomes well known for his ability to interpret dreams. And remember this is hardly a new profession even for Joseph in 1800 B.C. As already noted, the Egyptians had a long history of professional dream interpreters and so did the Mesopotamians. Joseph, like his father, had jealous siblings and was sold into slavery, eventually ending up in a Pharaoh's prison. Even Joseph's problems with his siblings came from a dream that he had where his interpretation was that his brothers should honor him.

In Genesis 40–42, it was said that while in prison, Joseph interpreted the dreams of two of the Pharaoh's domestic staff, giving one a favorable interpretation and the other an ominous one. Although both dreams came true as Joseph had predicted, Joseph lingered in jail two more years until the Pharaoh had two dreams with similar themes. In Genesis 41, it is written:

> Now it came about in the morning that his [the Pharaoh's] spirit was troubled, so he sent and called for all the magicians of Egypt, and all its sages. And the Pharaoh told them his dreams, but there was no one who could interpret

them... The Pharaoh sent and called for Joseph, and they hurriedly brought him out of the dungeon. And the Pharaoh said to Joseph, 'I have had a dream but no one can interpret it; and I have heard it said about you, that you can interpret it.' Joseph then answered the Pharaoh, saying, 'It is not in me; God will give the Pharaoh a favorable answer.'

When the Pharaoh related the two dreams, Joseph said that they were one and the same. Joseph predicted seven years of abundance followed by seven years of famine. However, Joseph told the Pharaoh that by preparing ahead and storing grain from the years of abundance, Egypt could avoid a major disaster. Joseph interpreted the meaning of having two similar dreams as an indication that God had made his mind up and the matter was settled. There was no changing the future but one could prepare oneself accordingly.

The Jewish religion shares with Christians the first five books of the Old Testament, collectively known as the Torah. The Talmud is a comprehensive book of Jewish laws, compiled between about 500 B.C. and A.D. 300. In it there are 217 references to dreams including one of the oldest recurring dreams, the loss of teeth. A professional dream interpreter in the Talmud was asked to interpret the loss of teeth in dreams. He offered the explanation that the dream portended death.

Dream references in the New Testament

In the New Testament, there are numerous references to dreams, particularly in Matthew. In Matthew 1, we are told Mary was found already to be pregnant although engaged to Joseph. It was said that Joseph was a righteous man but troubled by this event and thought about discreetly hiding Mary. In Matthew 1:19–21, it is written:

> But when he [Joseph] had considered this, behold, an angel of the Lord appeared to him in a dream, saying: 'Joseph, son of David, do not be afraid to take Mary as your wife; for that which has been conceived in her is of the Holy Spirit. And she will bear him a Son; and you shall call His name Jesus...'

In Matthew 2, it is written that three wise men from the east had sought out Mary and the baby Jesus, and finding them, they knelt down and paid Jesus homage. In Matthew 2:12, it is written that they were warned in a dream not to return to the evil King Herod who was also seeking Jesus. In Matthew 2:13, it is reported that another angel of the Lord appeared to Joseph in a dream and told him to flee with his family to Egypt, because Herod wished to kill Jesus. In Matthew 2:19, it is said that when Herod died, an angel again appeared to Joseph in a dream while in Egypt and told him to return to the land of Israel. Later, in verse 22, Joseph is said to be warned again in a dream, and he left for the district of Galilee.

It is also interesting to note that not only the beginning of Jesus' life was replete with divine information dreams and dream warnings, but the end of Jesus' life also involved dreams. Jesus was arrested by the local governor, Pontius Pilate, and while a captive, Matthew 27:19 reads:

> And while he [Pilate] was sitting on the judgment seat, his wife sent to him, saying, 'Have nothing to do with that righteous Man; for last night I suffered greatly in a dream because of Him.'

Pilate was obviously affected by his wife's dream (perhaps the first clear Biblical reference to a nightmare), washed his hands in front of the crowd, and declared himself innocent of the eventual spilling of Jesus' blood.

Later, Christians would also be influenced by their dreams. Most notable among them is the story of Joan of Arc (1412–1431), a French heroine, who reported having dream visions at the age of 13. She claimed that saints would talk to her, and she said that they told her that she was chosen to defeat the English in battle – which she then did! – although without a sufficient army. She was eventually defeated. In an interesting test of whether one should obey the church or the saints of God; she chose the latter, was convicted of blasphemy and burned to death at the stake. Twenty-five years later, she was legally declared innocent.

Greek Dream interpretation: the *Oneirocritica*

In the middle of the second century AD, Artemidorus, a Greek philosopher, published five books about dream interpretation known as the *Oneirocritica* (translation: *Interpretation of Dreams*) (Artemidorus, 1975). Interestingly, the last two books were written in letter form to his eponymously named son, an apprentice dream interpreter. Perhaps, with the exception of Freud's *Interpretation of Dreams*, the *Oneirocritica* has been the most quoted book on dream interpretation in history. Artemidorus attempted to offer his readers a system and principles for categorizing and interpreting dreams. Clearly, his work tapped into a long history of prior Grecian dream interpretation. Many of these works Artemidorus cited in his book, but there are few remaining copies of the earlier works.

Like his predecessors, Artemidorus argued that the dreamer's occupation, habits, and attitudes must all be taken into account before any dream could be interpreted. It is, perhaps, the most outstanding feature of the *Oneirocritica* that Artemidorus attempted to stay rational and practical in the interpretation of dreams and to eliminate prior influences of superstition and mysticism. Many of the roots of Freud's dream interpretation principles can be found in Artemidorus' work. For example, Artemidorus noted that many dreams are simply a continuation of the prior day's activities. He also noted that bodily needs or recent important events can be represented directly in a dream. Artemidorus argued that the age and health status of a person must be known before a dream could be interpreted. It appears that Artemidorus meant for the first three books to be read by the general public. The last two books were much more personal, and he even encouraged his son to keep the last two books private. They are both full of fatherly warnings and advice. He encouraged his son to fully learn the local customs and peculiarities of every place that his son traveled, not just for the sake of dream interpretation, but also to be a better person. Artemidorus argued that bad dreams seem to come true more quickly than good dreams, and he warned against mystical approaches to dreams, which he thought tended to attribute too much importance to inconsequential aspects of dreams. Like the modern dream interpreter, Fritz Perls, but 1800 years earlier, Artemidorus thought recurrent dreams were especially important.

Despite the many influential and practical aspects of Artemidorus' approach, he still reinforced a very long history of propounding a glossary of dream meanings. For example, to dream of a beard was interpreted by Artemidorus as a good omen. If a woman dreamed she had a beard and if she was a widow, it meant that she would marry again. If she already had a husband, then she would be separated from him. He also had an elaborate interpretation of tooth dreams, including very specific interpretations of the mouth, its right side and left side, molars, incisors, grinders, and canine teeth. The loss of teeth, either singly, together, or broken, Artemidorus interpreted as related to the payment of debts. Interestingly, if a sick person had the tooth loss dream, he thought it indicated a lingering illness but 'clearly signifies that no death will result.' The *Oneirocritica* also had long sections about the interpretation of sexual dreams; however, again these interpretations were all based on a glossary of meanings.

Later Jewish dream interpretation: the *Pitron Chalomot*

In Freud's book, *The Interpretation of Dreams,* he mentioned that Jewish dream interpretation may date to a book, *Dream Interpretation (Pitron Chalomot),* written by Almori in 1848. Apparently, Freud was unaware that the first edition of Almori's book occurred over 330 years earlier in 1515 in Constantinople. Furthermore, Jewish dream interpretation, as noted previously, had a far older history, with numerous dream references in both the Torah and the Talmud.

Almori was a Jewish Rabbi, judge, physician, and philosopher. At about the age of 30 in 1515, he published the book *Mefasher Chelmin (Dream Mediator),* which was later published as *Interpretation of Dreams (Pitron Chalomot).* Interestingly, he believed that everyone had at least one great thing to say in his or her lifetime. The book's success is relatively obvious, because Freud became aware of a copy printed over three centuries later, and a Yiddish version was printed as late as 1902 in Brooklyn, New York.

The *Pitron Chalomot* contains three sections: Almori's theory and principles of dream interpretation, a dictionary offering the interpretation of various dream symbols, and a discussion of the ways to 'break the spell' of bad dreams through religious rituals. The first section drew upon dream references in the Torah and the Talmud, as well as two other Jewish books, the Zohar and the Midrash. Almori began with the premise that it is a basic desire of people to understand the meaning of life. However, he firmly believed that, by virtue of people's very nature, they were incapable of this understanding, and thus required God's help. His primary idea was that this understanding could be acquired through the interpretation of dreams, and yet Almori believed even this avenue was fraught with difficulties. People were not practiced in the interpretation of dreams, and often they feared the meanings of their dreams, as well as fearing those who professed to be able to interpret their dreams. In Job 33:13–17, Elihu states that God opens the ears of men while they are sleeping, and yet they do not understand His decrees.

Almori decried the fact that dream interpretation had such a low status in contemporary society, and he felt strongly that dreams were not mere metaphors. He thought that dreams had consequence and that they could be divinely inspired, offering humanity a glimpse of the mind and purpose of God in their lives. He wrote:

> ...I, Solomon Almori, the most insignificant of my generation, became imbued with zeal for God, the God of prophets and of His people Israel, in order that His communications should not be lost. I took it upon myself to seek out every word written upon this subject [dreams] and then to transcribe these sayings, together with my own meager contributions, into a single small text that will bloom like a rose... I have titled this book 'Dream Mediator,' for I will set forth universally valid principles whereby all people will be able to interpret their dreams and understand their significance.
> (Covitz, 1990, p. 13).

In the first section of his book, Almori listed the hierarchical levels of dreams, the highest being the prophetic dream, and he gave the examples of prophetic dreams from the Torah of Jacob, Daniel, and Solomon. Jacob, for example, had the now legendary dream of angels ascending and descending a ladder suspended between heaven and earth. In the dream, God told him that he and his descendants would prosper (Genesis 28:13–14). With regard to prophetic dreams, Almori agreed with Aristotle, who believed that they could only come to the distinguished, wise, and powerful. Almori also believed that, unlike ordinary dreams (the second level of dreams), prophetic dreams had virtually no useless material in them.

For ordinary dreams, Almori gave the example of Joseph and the Pharaoh's dreams of an impending drought (Genesis 40–41). Almori noted that even ordinary dreams were one-sixtieth prophetic. The third level of dreams was the dreams of sorcerers and false prophets. Almori gave the example from Deuteronomy 13:2 that warns against the interpretations of dream-diviners, who could conjure the dream images they desired by preparing themselves before sleep to have particular images. In this case, Almori appears to have been describing what is now known as lucid dreaming (LaBerge, 1985), i.e. the ability of some people to become aware that they are dreaming and to affect the outcome of their dreams by preparing themselves before sleep.

Interestingly, in Almori's summary about his three levels of dreaming, he noted that it is an imperfect world, such that every dream will have some useless material, even prophetic dreams, but, more importantly, Almori claimed that 'you will never come across a dream that is totally without value... If we think a dream has no significance, we may be sure that we have failed to understand the dream' (Covitz, 1990, p.17). Almori also believed that it was the task of the dream interpreter to weed out the mundane and inconsequential aspects of a dream from the meaningful aspects. To support this contention, Almori cited the Talmud, where Rabbi Berakhiah stated that part of a dream may be fulfilled, but the whole of a dream can never be fulfilled.

Almori offers some additional dream interpretation principles, amazingly modern and useful. He again cites the Talmud: 'A dream that is not interpreted is like a letter that is not read.' Almori interprets this passage as a responsibility of the dreamer to have his or her dreams interpreted. Almori reasons that a dream cannot be fulfilled, for good or ill, if the dreamer does not have it interpreted. Almori also believed in the Talmudic passage that 'all dreams follow the mouth.' This arcane saying may have indicated that dream interpreters in the Talmud had some liberty in putting a positive spin on negative dreams, and even a negative spin on positive dreams. Thus an ancient, ethical dream interpreter, according to Almori, could have made positive outcomes from evil dreams, and vice versa. And what were the consequences of uninterpreted dreams? Almori strongly believed in the divine nature of dreams. He believed that if the dreamer failed to correctly understand the dream or failed to perform whatever was required of the dreamer, God would no longer communicate anything important to the dreamer, and all dreams would become inconsequential and insignificant.

An overall summary of Almori's dream interpretation techniques is amazingly contemporary. The modern dream interpreter Ernest Hartmann, as noted in Chapter 1, appears not so much an innovator in light of Almori's work, as a rediscoverer of Almori's dream principles. Like Hartmann, Almori believed that dreams communicate messages using a metaphor or an allegory. Almori also noted that two people may have the same dream, and the interpretation could be quite different. He noted that every dreamer could derive a different interpretation from the same dream based on his or her unique past and different personality. He also noted that dream interpretation was dependent upon wisdom, and therefore not everyone could readily interpret dreams.

Buddhists

Dreams also played a central role in the story of the founding of Buddhism:

> In 544 B.C., Buddha's future mother, queen Maha-Maya, was at a feast. After eating, she returned to her royal couch and had the following dream.
>
> Four guardian angels came and lifted her up, together with her couch, and took her away to the Himalayan Mountains. There...they laid her under a prodigious sal-tree. Then came the wives of these guardian angels, and conducted her to Anotatta Lake, and bathed her, to remove every human stain... Not far off was Silver Hill, and in it a golden mansion. There they spread a divine couch with its head towards the east, and laid her down upon it. Now the Future Buddha had become a superb white elephant, and was wandering about at no great distance, on Gold Hill. Descending thence, he ascended Silver Hill, and approaching from the north, he plucked a white lotus with his silvery trunk, and trumpeting loudly, went into the golden mansion. And three times he walked round his mother's couch, with his right side towards it, and striking her on her right side he seemed to enter her womb. Thus the conception took place in the Midsummer Festival.
>
> On the next day the queen awoke, and told the dream to the king. And the king caused 64 eminent Brahmans to be summoned, and spread costly seats for them on ground festively prepared with green leaves, Dalbergia flowers, and so forth. The Brahmans being seated... And when their every desire had been satisfied, he told them the dream and asked them what would come of it.
>
> 'Be not anxious, great king!' said the Brahmans; 'a great child has planted itself in the womb of your queen, and it is a male child not a female. You will have a son. And he, if he continue to live the household life, will become a Universal Monarch; but if he leave the household life and retire from the world, he will become a Buddha, and roll back the clouds of sin and folly of this world.'
> (de Becker, 1968; p. 42–5)

Interestingly, this virginal conception predates by 500 years the Christian belief that Christ was conceived without sexual intercourse. And perhaps more amazing is that Joseph, the stepfather of Jesus, is made aware of Jesus' conception in the exact same way as Buddha's mother – from a dream.

Hindus

The Hindu religion has no single sacred text, yet there is a sacred core of works, and in all of them there are references to dreams. The oldest of these sacred books are the Vedas, which are thought to have been written from about 1500 B.C. to 1000 B.C. The Vedas contain not only interpretations of dreams much like the

Egyptians', where particular activities or symbols are given either a favorable or unfavorable prognosis, but also the Vedas offer rather sophisticated theories for the role that dreams play in unconscious and conscious daily waking life. The archetypal dream of the loss of teeth is also present, predating the Talmudic reference by at least 1000 years, and, as in the Talmud, it has ominous and foreboding meaning for the dreamer.

A second major religious Indian treatise is the Upanishads, which were written from about 900 B.C. to about 500 B.C., and they also contain references to dreams. The Bhradaranyaka Upanishad offers two theories of dreaming. One is similar to the Freudian notion that all of the objects in a dream actually represent the dreamer's secret wishes and desires. The second theory is similar to a Chinese dream idea that the soul wanders about during dream sleep, and that if a dreamer is suddenly awakened their soul may not have time to return to its body and the dreamer might die. The last three holy Hindu works are the Ramayana, Mahabharata, and the Bhagavad Gita (actually a part of the Mahabharata). They were written about the same time as the Talmud, about 300 B.C. to A.D. 200. All three of these sacred works contains references to dreams, particularly prophetic dreams.

Chinese texts

One of the classic texts in Chinese history is the *T'ung Shu* (1986), translation: *Book of Myriad Things*. The core history of the *T'ung Shu* dates back well over 4000 years, and it was initially created as an almanac, commissioned by Chinese rulers, giving details of the lunar calendar and the seasons. Subsequent additions to the annual production of the *T'ung Shu* consisted of advice and essays on geomancy (feng shui), herbal medicines and cures, fortune telling, numerology, legends, predictions, and even pregnancy charts. In approximately 1000 B.C., a new section was added to the *T'ung Shu* entitled 'Old Mr Chou's Book of Auspicious and Inauspicious Dreams.' Mr Chou was reputed to have been a reference to Chou Kung, the Duke of Chou, who may have assisted in the compilation of the *I Ching*, one of the most important Chinese works of divination. Even in modern times, the link remains between Old Mr Chou's name and dreams. For example, a teacher who encounters a sleeping student might say, 'Are you visiting Mr Chou?'

The similarities to the ancient Egyptians' dream writings are striking. Both texts listed dreams as good and bad, auspicious and inauspicious, and both employed puns, although some of the latter are lost through the vagaries of time and translation. Also, there have been recorded dreams in both cultures in which an emperor divined their future authority and ruled through a dream. It is also important to note that classic and ancient Chinese texts did not rely solely on dreams for divination because the Chinese had other means of foretelling the future, such as the zodiacal predictions, geomancy (feng shui), palmistry, numerology, physiognomy, charms, talismans, etc. Interestingly both cultures' dream texts noted dreams of civil and criminal legal actions regarding the dreamer.

Old Mr Chou's Book of Dreams in the *T'ung Shu* is divided into seven categories and examples of each category follow:

1   The Heavens and the Weather.
    If you dream of the sun or moon rising, then your family will prosper.
    If you dream of a dark, cloudy, drizzly day, then someone is going to die or be killed.
2   Features such as Houses, Gardens, Forests, etc.
    If you dream of lying on a large stone, then you will have good fortune.
    If you dream of an empty town, then you could be murdered.
3   Gods, Fairies, Spirits, etc.
    If you dream of visiting a temple, then you will have extremely good fortune.
    If you dream of a dead person rising from a coffin, you will earn a lot of money.
4   The Human Body.
    Dreaming of your teeth falling out means your parents are in danger.
    Dreams of growing teeth means that you will have many sons and grand-sons.
5   Being Out of Harmony with Someone – Music.
    To dream that you or anyone kills a duck, goose, or chicken means very good fortune.
    To dream of killing a lamb is a sign of evil or danger.
6   Living Creatures, Birds, Animals, etc.
    If you dream that a snake bites you, it means lots of money.
    If you dream of any bird flying into your house, it means that you will soon come into danger.
7   Clothing, Jewelry, and Miscellaneous Items.
    To dream of a fish breaking a boat implies bad fortune.
    To dream of picking up money is good fortune.

There are some other references to dreams in ancient Chinese literature, such as in the writings of Confucius. Compared with other ancient cultures, it may be surmised that the Chinese also relied upon dreams as a source of revelation and that they also had additional bases on which to divine and foretell the future other than dreams.

Islamic religion

The Prophet Muhammad (570–632), founder of the Muslim religion, had his first vision (or dream – apparently the written accounts of the event varies) at the age of 40, when the angel Gabriel appeared to him when he was alone meditating in the mountains near Mecca. He went home fearfully to tell his wife because he believed that he might have gone insane. She reassured him of his goodness but took him to a Christian cousin who listened to the angel's revelations to Muhammad. The cousin said that the revelations were the truth and the same teachings as brought by Moses and Jesus (e.g. Dawood, 1956). There is some consensus among contemporary Islamic scholars that the interpretation of dreams and divine dreams are gifts bestowed on whom Allah wills.

Mormon religion

Joseph Smith (1805–1844), the founder of the Mormon religion, or Church of the Latter-Day Saints, was an unschooled boy of 14 when he reported his first dream vision of God and Jesus Christ. At 22, the angel Moroni was said to have appeared to Smith and gave him the Egyptian-like characters on golden plates. Smith translated the script into the Book of Mormon and quickly attracted many followers for his new religion. Early in 1844, Smith declared his candidacy for the U.S. presidency. However, in June of 1844, a mob of angry Mormon dissidents swarmed the jail where Smith and his brother were held for destroying the dissidents' newspaper press, and they were murdered. Today, the Mormon religion is predominant in the state of Utah and is known throughout the world for its missionary work.

Final thoughts

It is no small irony that the world's cultural and religious history has been so intimately influenced by dream communications with God. Yet modern history, particularly the twentieth and early twenty-first centuries, has been characterized by a nearly complete absence of reports of people's dream communications with God. In fact, dreams of communication with God are generally dismissed as invalid or the product of deranged minds.

Jung pondered this question of why people complained that God no longer speaks to them like He used to. He thought that members of contemporary society got too tangled up in their own conscious worlds and had forgotten that God spoke primarily through dreams and visions. On the difference between dreams and visions, Jung viewed them both as emanating from the unconscious. The main difference to Jung appeared trivial: visions occurred only in the waking state.

Jung argued that whatever the unconscious might ultimately prove to be, there was no denying that it was a natural phenomenon that produced meaningful symbols. Jung asked any rational theologian: 'By what authority does he suggest that God is unable to speak through dreams?' Furthermore, Christian doctrine even states that some concepts, like the Holy Trinity, can only be understood through divine revelation.

So when people complained and asked why it was that God no longer talked to them, Jung said it reminded him of the rabbi who was asked the same question and who replied: 'Nowadays there is no longer anybody who can bow low enough.'

Summary

1 The earliest history of dream interpretation dates back at least 4000 years and has an interesting and repeating theme: communication between God and people through dreams.
2 The early Mesopotamians (about 2000 B.C.) had a rich history of dream interpretation including the practice of dream incubation.
3 The Egyptians were thought to have been influenced by the Mesopotamians, and they recorded hundreds of dreams and their interpretation on papyrus.
4 Early Jewish and Christian (200 B.C.–A.D. 300) writings, including the Torah and Talmud, and both testaments of the Bible, are replete with dream and dream interpretation references.
5 In the middle of the second century A.D., Artemidorus, a Greek philosopher, published a compilation of writings about dream interpretation. The book was called the *Oneirocritica*, and it has been one of the most quoted books on dream interpretation in history.
6 A Jewish rabbi and dream interpreter, Almori, published the Pitron Chalomot (translation: Dream Interpretation) in 1515. It contained many ancient and still current notions about dream interpretation including the idea that dreams can provide greater meaning to our lives.
7 Buddhist writings also contain references to dreams, including the story of the conception of Buddha by himself in the form of a white elephant.
8 Hindu sacred works also contain references, including the roles that dreams may play in our waking conscious lives.
9 Early Chinese texts (approximately 4000 years ago) also have references to dreams, and the tradition of dream interpretation is recorded in the *T'ung Shu*.
10 Islamic scholars credit a divine vision or dream bestowed by Allah upon the Prophet Muhammad in about A.D. 600 for the founding of the Muslim religion.
11 Joseph Smith, founder of the Mormon religion in about A.D. 1830, credits a divine vision or dream from the angel Moroni for his creation of the Book of Mormon.

CHAPTER 4

A triune model for sleep and dreams

At the end of Chapter 2, I established the fact that it is very difficult to awaken people from slow-wave sleep. I also noted that REM sleep is accompanied by muscle atonia (muscle paralysis). Thus the chapter ended with a paradox: sleeping on the ground, while it may have released early human types to receive more deep sleep (delta waves) and REM sleep, made them much more susceptible to ending up as a predator's dinner. In this chapter, I will present three major advantages (a triune model) that sleeping on the ground may have provided which outweighed the dangers. However, I will initially cover some other theorists' speculations as to the reasons we sleep and dream, as a background to my own.

The Hobson and McCarley activation-synthesis hypothesis

In 1977, Hobson and McCarley proposed a neurophysiological explanation for REM sleep. They called their model an *activation-synthesis hypothesis* which proposed that dreams do indeed represent an active model of the brain during sleep; however, this activation is not necessarily evolutionarily advantageous; in fact, they said, dreams are essentially meaningless and random. They proposed that an area of the brainstem known as the pons gives rise to electrical spikes that create REM sleep by randomly stimulating the areas of the brain above the brainstem (called the forebrain). These spikes begin in the pons, continue to the lateral geniculate nucleus, and then finally reach the visual cortex (occipital lobes). Thus the spikes are called PGO spikes, for pons-geniculate-occipital. When the forebrain is confronted by the resulting bizarre array of random visions and thoughts, it attempts to synthesize them into a coherent or semi-coherent story. However, because the storm of pontine spikes has randomly stimulated the forebrain, dreams usually end up more likely to be semi-coherent or even incoherent and full of distortion.

The Hobson and McCarley hypothesis was provocative (which is one of the purposes of a good theory) but it served up a storm of protests. In fact, I had a vivid dream about this time where I dreamt I was wandering the halls of a research hospital, the walls and floors of which were lined with soft mashed potatoes. As I saw myself walking through the mushy hallways, I knew in the dream that this was a ridiculous concept, but I trudged through the halls nonetheless. The opponents to their theory argued that even if it was pontine spikes that stimulated cortical thoughts, there still might be valid and, perhaps, hidden reasons for what people ultimately dream about. For example, I might be stimulated to dream about hospitals and mashed potatoes, whereas a former colleague of mine told me she dreamt of a Vietnamese frog without legs. Hospitals and mashed potatoes are in my cortex, and Vietnamese frogs without legs are in her cortex. I did not dream her dream, nor she mine. My intuition tells me that our choices, although strange and bizarre, are still not random. Hobson and McCarley's theory does provide a physiological explanation for REM sleep and an explanation for the seemingly bizarre or incoherent content of dreams. However, it fails miserably as an informal test of intuition: that is, does it seem at all reasonable, given all of our own experiences with dreaming, that dreams are meaningless? I don't think so.

By 1988, Hobson had tempered his original views about the meaninglessness of dreams. In his book *The Dreaming Brain*, he proposed that dreams do actually provide clear and meaningful themes along with conflictual issues that may be of value to the dreamer. He agreed with Jung that dreams have transparent meaning, and he disagreed with Freud that dreams have a latent or hidden meaning. In his 1994 book, *The Chemistry of Conscious States*, he carried his analysis of dreams even further by likening dream states to mental illnesses. For example, he saw the anxiety caused by nightmares as similar to panic disorders, the visual images in our dreams as similar to visual hallucinations that occur in psychoses, and the poor memory that we have about our dreams as akin to the forgetting that occurs in Alzheimer's disease. In fact, Hobson argued even more strongly that dreams are not models of mental illness. He said, 'Dreaming is not a *model* of a psychosis. It *is* a psychosis. It's just a healthy one.' Thus Hobson argued that understanding the 'root cause' of dreaming will help us to understand the 'genesis' of psychotic states. He also provided an analysis of dreams by means of a mental status examination, which is a short intake interview upon admission to a hospital to establish a patient's general cognitive functioning. To me, it was weakly argued and a poor analogy. However, it is interesting to note that Hobson was reinforcing Wundt's (1896) much older view of dreaming as a kind of hallucinatory insanity and that dreams gave us a view of what a mental disturbance would be like.

Winson's memory-processing hypothesis

Winson (1990) has established that a *theta rhythm* of 6 Hz arises from the hippocampus of awake animals in specific and important functions, such as exploratory behavior in rats, a fear response resulting in rigidity in rabbits, and predation in cats. Furthermore, these behaviors are not rigidly genetically encoded like feeding and procreation, but occur in response to changing environmental circumstances. Because the role of the hippocampus has been well documented in establishing the permanence of memory in both people and animals, he reasoned that the theta rhythm might be the cause of permanent memory transformations. He also found the same theta rhythm in REM sleep in rats, and the same neurons of the hippocampus fired during REM sleep that had fired while the rats were awake and learning a maze. Because exploratory behavior in rats appears critical to their survival, Winson argued that the purpose of REM sleep might be to process and strengthen this critical information.

Winson offers another line of evidence for his theory from evolution. The spiny anteater is a unique egg-laying mammal (called a monotreme). The spiny anteater does not have REM sleep and appeared to diverge from other mammals like marsupials and placentals about 140 million years ago. The spiny anteater also has the largest prefrontal cortex in relation to the rest of its brain of any mammal, even people. Winson argues that the spiny anteater needs this large prefrontal cortex to store new and crucial information and to be able to make decisions based on previously stored information. However, in order to develop even more sophisticated capabilities, a new storage mechanism is needed beyond that of simply adding more space (like increasing the size of the cortex). Thus, he stated:

> REM sleep could have provided this new mechanism, allowing memory processing to occur 'off-line.' Coincident with the apparent development of REM sleep in marsupial and placental animals was a remarkable neuroanatomical change: the prefrontal cortex was dramatically reduced in size. Far less prefrontal cortex was required to process information. That area of the brain could then develop to provide advanced perceptual and cognitive abilities in higher species.
>
> With the evolution of REM sleep, each species could process the information most important for its survival, such as the location of food or the means of predation or escape – those activities during which theta rhythm is present. In REM sleep this information may be accessed again and integrated with past experience to provide an ongoing strategy for behavior.
>
> Dreams may reflect a memory-processing mechanism inherited from lower species, in which information important for survival is reprocessed during REM sleep.

Winson's theory is provocative and compelling. It does not, however, adequately take into account why infants and children spend 50% of their time in REM sleep nor why after the age of about two years REM sleep remains constant across the lifespan. Furthermore, the same theta rhythm of hippocampal origin has not been found in humans or any other primates, to date.

A triune sleep model

In the chapter on Freud in this book, I will describe his notion that dream elements are overdetermined, that is, dreams have more than one meaning. I am proposing a similar notion for why slow-wave and REM sleep have developed. I believe that they developed for more than one reason, and thus part of the problem for developing a good reason for sleep has been impeded by the logical structure imposed by some researchers that a good etiological theory of sleep mutually excludes other theories. Here is my triune theory.

Recuperative value of sleep

One function of sleep appears to be that it is restorative or recuperative. Hess (1954) also described this process as reparative and argued that this must be the vital function of sleep because sleep renders an organism so helpless for a large part of each 24-hour epoch. Thus, one element of sleep as a restorative process is that the organism not only protects itself from wearing out but it also builds its energy resources back up during sleep. The organism 'needs' rest because its store of energy is depleted. This need for rest is hypothesized to be instinctual, inherited, and evolutionarily adaptive.

First, it is a curious phenomenon that most modern researchers (like Webb, 1975) make the restorative versus any-other-reason-for-sleep theory 'either/or' propositions. As the ethologist Gould (1985; 1986) has noted evolution is not directed by a 'perfect architect.' The process of natural selection results in dead ends, 'odd solutions,' and 'imperfections.' He wrote that 'adaptations...[are] jerry-rigged from parts available.' The Yale psychiatrist Reiser (1990) argued that 'REM sleep was just such an available part.' He wrote:

> ...I propose that the mind exploits the unique REM brain state for its own purposes, so to speak. This view accords *prior* biologic significance to the REM state. The assumption is that REM sleep appeared first in the course of evolutionary mammalian development and, favoring survival, was retained and further developed. [...] The anatomic/physiologic patterns of brain circuitry in the REM state of the brain...are of such a nature that they can also subserve patterns and mechanisms of perceptual and memory processing, that, also favoring survival, were retained and further developed and that acquired adaptive importance of their own. [italics mine]

Thus Reiser's argument supports my initial premise that sleep and REM may be overdetermined, and his argument at least allows for the coexistence of recuperative and other theories for sleep because sleep and REM may have had prior biologic significance. Psychobiologist Beatty (1995) has written of an energy balance, referring to 'the relationship between energy intake in the form of food and energy outflow or expenditure.' Continuous motion over 24-hour cycles would have required nearly continuous foraging and hunting. People presently do not have the energy to be on the go 24 hours a day. Thus we have evolved from ancestors who did have limited energy, enough, perhaps, for 16 to 19 hours of activity. After this period, the organism would indeed have been exhausted.

There are at least two other pieces of evidence for a recuperative theory. First, it is interesting that during stage 4 sleep, the parasympathetic system predominates. This part of the autonomic nervous system controls vegetative functions like the digestive and gastrointestinal systems, which become highly active during stage 4. Apparently in order to aid these processes and further conserve energy, the cardiovascular system becomes slower, and heart rate, blood pressure, and respiration all decrease. These active digestive and gastrointestinal processes result in the production of more energy and the expulsion of waste products. Most people, in all cultures, excrete in the morning upon awakening, and curiously, feel refreshed with the energy to face another day.

My second piece of evidence comes from REM sleep. Again, continuous muscle activity would require enormous amounts of food to be converted into energy. A person continuously on the go would have had to develop some period where the blood and oxygen supply would be temporarily diverted for digestion. Not only that, these muscles would have to be extraordinary in their ability to keep firing without rest. Yet we know that even our remotest ancestors were not capable of continuous sustained motion. Muscles have a refractory period where it is hypothesized that they recuperate from their labors, and it may be that there are micro-refractory periods (brief rest after short exertions) and macro-refractory periods (like long periods of sleep). This notion of activity and rest is also consistent with a theory in psychology (based on a physics theory) called opponent process, which states that for every action there is an opposite reaction. Interestingly, REM sleep is accompanied by complete skeletal muscle relaxation, nearly two full hours a night of deep muscle relaxation. At least anecdotally, body builders will tell you that a muscle cannot build itself up without regular periods of rest after exercise, and they say that overtraining is almost as bad as undertraining in terms of muscle development.

Even if these arguments fall on unsympathetic ears, I would strongly argue with the necessity of a single theory. There is mounting evidence that sleep and REM may presently serve far more than a single function. In addition, the purposes of non-REM and REM appear to change not only phylogenetically but also ontologically. For example, the amount of stage 4 sleep decreases dramatically to nearly zero after about the age of 65. Whatever purpose stage 4 sleep serves when we are younger, it appears to lose this purpose when we are older. And is there a concomitant loss of behavioral function with the loss of stage 4? As for REM, it has been hypothesized that REM sleep plays an important role in developing, programming, and stimulating the maturation of the infant brain, even in utero. In older people, what functions of REM sleep remain, if any, of the earlier functions of REM?

A third piece of evidence comes from Pinel (1993) who helped advance a sophisticated variant of the adaptive model of sleep, circadian theory. According to Pinel:

> Circadian theories argue that sleep is not a response to internal balance...a neural mechanism has evolved to encourage animals to sleep during those times of the day when they do not usually engage in activities necessary for their survival...and their strong motivation to sleep at night may have evolved to conserve their energy resources and to make them less susceptible to mishap (e.g. predation) in the dark. The circadian theory views sleep as an instinct somewhat akin to the instinct to engage in sexual activity...the circadian theories regard sleep as a strict parent who demands inactivity because it keeps us out of trouble.

Actually, it can be argued that the neurobiochemistry of non-REM and REM sleep suggests that they are a clear function of internal balance. Nonetheless, Pinel noted that while circadian theories account for the results of sleep deprivation studies better than recuperative studies, 'it is not necessarily an all-or-none issue; recuperative models and circadian models are not mutually exclusive.'

A final piece of evidence for the recuperative power of sleep comes from the following doctor:

> At the fork of a road
> In the Vale of Va-vode
> Five foot-weary salesmen have laid down their load.
> All day they've raced round in the heat, at top speeds,
> Unsuccessfully trying to sell Zizzer-Zoof Seeds
> Which nobody wants because nobody needs.
> Tomorrow will come. They'll go back to their chore.
> They'll start on the road, Zizzer-Zoofing once more
> But tonight they've forgotten their feet are so sore.
> And that's what the wonderful night time is for.
> Geisel, 1962, from *Dr. Seuss's Sleep Book*

Adaptive value: priming and creativity

Priming

Priming is said to have occurred when recognition or performance is facilitated by prior exposure to the target stimuli. I propose that the content of REM sleep, and, perhaps, thoughts and ideas from other stages, may serve to prime sleepers to be response-ready in their subsequent waking activities. For example, imagine two ancient hunters, the night before a big hunt. One dreams he (or she) has forgotten to bring his (or her) extra knife on the hunt. The other dreams away blissfully. In the morning, the anxious dreamer is prompted to remember his or her extra knife upon awakening. The other dreamer forgets the extra knife. Who is more likely to survive and adapt should an extra knife be needed? I think it would be the anxious dreamer. Thus, the anxious content of our dreams can prime us to be more successful in our waking life.

Freud (1900/1956) noted at least two dreams that may have had ancient ancestral roots: (i) the examination dream, and (ii) the embarrassment of being naked dream. In both instances, the dreams may serve to prime the dreamer to be prepared in his or her subsequent waking life. In the examination dream, the dreamer is unprepared for an examination about to be undertaken. Freud noted that the dream may appear years after any actual examinations may have been taken and that they may represent neurotic (anxiety) fears of being punished for being unprepared by our parents or schoolmasters. Freud interpreted the dreams of being naked or partially clothed as repressed sexual wishes. It is possible that both dreams had their origins in the ancestral hominoid (about 2 million years ago) environment. Hunters who were improperly dressed for hunting might die in a sudden and harsh weather change. Hunters without proper stone tools or weapons might also regret their lack of preparedness. The replay of these themes may have served to prime the dreamers so that they were less likely actually to commit these errors upon awakening.

Revonsuo (2000) has proposed a *threat simulation theory*, which states that the present dream-production system simulates threatening events in the ancestral environment. Revonsuo offers two major lines of evidence, common dreams of children, adolescents, and adults, and dreams of contemporary hunter-gatherers.

Van de Castle (1983) and Domhoff (1996), in large surveys of children's dream reports, found that animal characters made up the largest proportion of children's dreams (approximately 20–45%). They noted that the animals in dreams tended to be those that were rarely, if ever, encountered in children's actual lives, e.g. monsters, bears, wolves, snakes, gorillas, tigers, lions, and biting insects. The authors also noted that college students and older individuals, whose percentage of animal dreams was much lower, tended to dream of animals more likely to be encountered in real life, e.g. horses, dogs, and cats. Children's dreams also had higher rates of aggression than adult dreams, and higher rates of aggression involving animals. Actually, children do dream of common animals but that fact does not necessarily negate Revonsuo's hypothesis.

The recurrent dreams of adults, in particular nightmares, may also present a glimpse of ancestral dream life. Robbins and Houshi (1983), in a study of college students, reported that the most common recurring dream theme was anxiety in the context of being pursued or threatened. The most common themes in nightmares, of course, contain high levels of anxiety but also appear similar to recurrent dream themes such as being threatened, chased, or attacked.

Revonsuo (2000) argued that the waking lives of most of these dreamers, and especially children, were unlikely to have high levels of real daily threats, especially attacks by wild animals. He hypothesized that the dreamers were reliving archaic dream themes, particularly ones that would simulate the real dangers of the ancestral environment, including falling, violent encounters with natural disasters, and being threatened by strange people and wild animals. He reasoned that through natural selection, dreaming came to be a biological function that rehearsed threat perception and threat avoidance. The selective advantage would come from a dream theme repetition that would enhance and prepare waking threat-avoidance skills, which, as I noted earlier, is called priming.

There is evidence from the dream reports of contemporary hunter-gatherers that daily confrontations do increase dream themes of aggression and anxiety. Domhoff (1996) reported the results of dream studies conducted in the 1930s on Yir Yoront, a group of native Australian hunter-gatherers. The adult males had significantly higher percentages of dreams with animals, aggression involving animals, and physical aggression than did those of male American dreamers. Gregor (1977) analyzed the dreams of Mehinaku Indians of Central Brazil. He found significantly more aggression and animal-aggression themes than those of American dreamers. Gregor estimated that about 60% of the dreams of the Mehinaku males had threatening themes, while only 20% of their dreams involved nonthreatening or nonaggressive activities. In a classic study of one adult woman of the contemporary !Kung hunters-and-gatherers of the Kalahari desert, Shostak (1981) recorded over ten dreams with recurring and threatening themes of sexual infidelity, jealousy, omens, and divinations, and falling (while climbing a tree, and into a well). These findings are again consistent with my priming hypothesis and Revonsuo's threat simulation theory, and it appears highly probable that threatening ancestral environments helped sustain threatening dream themes in our earliest ancestors.

Creativity

Modern evidence for creativity and dreams is largely anecdotal but replete throughout the arts and sciences. Artists who claimed their work was based on a dream include Durer, Goya, Blake, Rousseau, Dali, and Magritte, among many others. Musicians who claimed a work was based on a dream include Mozart, Wagner, Keith Richards (lead guitarist for the Rolling Stones claimed the musical riff to '[I Can't Get No] Satisfaction' came in a dream), and Billy Joel, again among many others. The eighteenth century violinist Tartini reported that his inspiration for his most famous violin work, 'Trillo del Diavolo' (The Devil's Trill), came to him during a dream in which the devil played a particular violin riff. Upon awakening, he reported that he excitedly tried to duplicate the devil's trill. This story was also undoubtedly the inspiration for country-rock musician Charlie Daniels' fiddle song *The Devil Went Down to Georgia*.

A number of writers have claimed that the inspiration for a work came in a dream. Robert Louis Stevenson wrote that while pondering a duality that exists in all humans, he dreamt the story for Dr. Jekyll and Mr Hyde in virtually a single dream. Samuel Taylor Coleridge claimed that his poem 'Kubla Khan' came to him in a dream and that upon awakening he wrote down about 40 lines before he was interrupted by someone, and thus left the poem incomplete (in fairness, it is not known to what extent opium addictions may also have played a role in some anecdotal dream reports; *see* Hartmann, 1998 for more complete descriptions of creativity, dreaming and critiques).

Two chemists have anecdotally reported their most famous discoveries resulted from dreams. In the nineteenth century, the Russian chemist Dmitri Mendeleyev said he conceived of the periodic table in a dream (Van de Castle, 1994). Also in the nineteenth century, German-born and later French chemist Friedrich Kekulé had been pondering the structure of the benzene molecule. He knew that it had six carbon atoms but neither a branching chain nor a straight alignment would account for its chemical properties. In a dream, he saw snake-like 'conformations' writhing together. He reported that one of the snakes had seized its own tail and 'whirled mockingly' before his eyes. He said he awoke in a 'flash of lightning,' and began working out his famous solution to the problem, the benzene ring. It has been suggested, however, that Kekulé may have made this claim to avoid accusations that he had borrowed his idea from the work of others (*see* Hartmann, 1998 for a more complete discussion). Again in the 1800s, American Elias Howe reported that he had worked for five years trying to create an automatic sewing machine. He said that he could not figure out how to get the machine to grab the thread once it had pierced the material. In his dream, he said he was a missionary captured by natives. They stood around him dancing with spears that had holes in their tips. Upon awakening, he said that he recognized this was the solution to his problem, a needle with a hole in the tip.

There is also a plethora of anecdotal reports of creative ideas and solutions for problems arising from dreams. For example, Krippner and Hughes (1970) found, in a survey of contemporary mathematicians, that over 50% reported they had at least once solved a mathematical problem in a dream. The brilliant Indian mathematician Ramanujan (1887–1920) said that the goddess Kali gave him solutions to theorems in his dreams, although there was some suspicion he said so for politico-religious reasons. There is also the phenomenon of lucid dreaming, where dreamers can become aware that they are dreaming within a dream, and thus control the direction or outcome of the dream. This technique has reportedly been used successfully as a psychotherapeutic technique, as claimed by its proponents (e.g. Cartwright and Lamberg, 1992; LaBerge, 1985). However, lucid dreams are infrequent, and few people can successfully and regularly control their dreams (e.g. Hartmann, 1998).

Is there a physiological mechanism that could account for the creative process in dreams? One such mechanism, as mentioned earlier, is well known: pons-geniculate-occipital (PGO) spikes. These electrical waves from the pons (in the brainstem), or PGO spikes, randomly stimulate the visual cortex by way of the lateral geniculate nucleus (part of the thalamus involved in vision). The resulting stimulation of the cortex results in visions and themes that may then be synthesized into a coherent story.

Hartmann (1998), as noted earlier, speculates that these dream stories allow the dreamer to make connections between disparate and often contradictory ideas. These connections, he proposes, are often more broad and inclusive than during wakefulness. By the nature of cognition, some intent and coherence is imposed and guided by the emotions (and limbic structures) of the dreamer. Thus Hartmann believes dreams contextualize emotions and, by using visual and spatial pathways, create an explanatory metaphor for the dreamer's emotional state. More importantly, Hartmann saw the process as allowing for new ideas and new ways of doing things, and he proposed that it allows the very important cognitive process of creating metaphors.

Whereas there exists a plethora of anecdotal evidence and personal speculation for the general claim that dreaming, problem solving, and creativity are linked, there have been few experimental attempts. Dement (1972) gave 500 undergraduates a problem to solve 15 minutes before sleeping. In the morning, they reported their dreams and any solution to the problem. Of 1148 attempts, it was reported that the solution came in a dream on only seven occasions (less than 1%). Blagrove (1992) presented a critique of problem solving in the dream literature and concluded that there is little empirical evidence that new and useful solutions to waking problems are created in dream sleep. He did propose that psychological solutions may be correlated with dreaming, but it did not imply a causative relationship. He counter-argued that solutions may more often occur while awake, and subsequent dreaming merely reflects the solution. In summary, there is no wealth of compelling experimental evidence for the link between creativity and dreams; however, the preponderance of anecdotal and other sources of evidence makes it a difficult hypothesis to dismiss completely, and a recent empirical study has certainly revived the idea.

In a study of sleep and creative problem solving, Wagner *et al.* (2004) gave 106 human participants a cognitive task that required learning stimulus-response sequences (which they deemed an implicit procedural memory task) where improvement, as measured by reaction time, was evident over trials. Participants could improve abruptly if they gained insight into a hidden abstract rule. After initial training, participants either slept for eight hours or stayed awake (at night or during the day) for a similar period. Twice as many participants who slept became aware of the hidden rule than those who stayed awake, regardless of time of day. Based on a slowing of reaction times in the sleep group, the authors postulated that the participants' greater insight was not a strengthening of the procedural memory itself but involved a novel restructuring of the original representations. They speculated that the restructuring was mediated by the hippocampus, related medial temporal lobe structures, and prefrontal cortex.

These structures have been previously shown to play an important role in generating awareness in memory. Wagner *et al.* suspected that cell assemblies representing newly learned tasks were reactivated by the hippocampal structures during sleep and incorporated by the neocortex into pre-existing long-term memories. They hypothesized that this process of incorporation into long-term storage formed the basis for the remodeling and qualitatively different restructuring of representations in memory. Thus, in their opinion, sleep may serve as a catalyst for insight.

Mnemonitive value: memory consolidation and enhancement

Consciousness is a continuum from awake to asleep. Wakefulness obviously varies from very aware to semi-aware (some freshmen in lectures), but sleep also varies in levels of awareness. Mentation is nearly entirely absent in the slow-wave sleep, but REM sleep often includes 'paradoxical awareness,' which is the state of being selectively aware of some aspects of our external sleeping environment (for example, muscle atony, or strange sounds or our names), yet sleeping through most other sounds and stimuli. Furthermore, we can become aware that we are dreaming, but more often than not, we accept our dream and our awareness of it as reality. Because learning and memory formation are aspects of consciousness (although there is some evidence for some types of learning without awareness), there is reason to suspect that memories are stabilized and consolidated during sleep, both slow-wave and REM. Indeed, it would not be reasonable to suspect that these activities would stop altogether during sleep, although it also seems plausible that these activities might be reduced during sleep (particularly active learning).

As mentioned previously, the first strong empirical research for REM's role in memory consolidation came from the work of Winson (1990). Winson found that theta rhythms in sleeping rats in their hippocampal neurons fired in similar patterns to their awake firing while learning mazes. Because exploratory behavior in rats appears critical to their survival, Winson reasoned one purpose of REM sleep might be the strengthening and consolidation of these visuospatial (procedural) memories.

General support for Winson's hypothesis comes from a gene study by Ribeiro *et al.* (1999). They studied the expression of a plasticity-associated gene, zif-268, during the slow-wave and REM sleep of rats that had been exposed to an enriched sensorimotor experience in a preceding waking period. They found that non-exposed control rats showed a generalized response in zif-268 during slow-wave and REM sleep, whereas the exposed rats showed upregulation in zif-268 during REM sleep in the hippocampus and cerebral cortex. They interpreted this finding as evidence that REM sleep opens a window of increased neural plasticity, presumably enhancing and/or consolidating the memory of the enriched experience.

The evidence for the enhancement of declarative memories (i.e. the memories for facts and verbal material) during the sleep of humans is far more controversial. For example, there is only minimal evidence for the ability to learn verbal material during sleep, and in any case it appears to be a highly inefficient method of learning (e.g. Levy, Coolidge, and Staab, 1972). Most studies that have found any positive effect of slow-wave or REM sleep upon declarative memories have used a sleep-stage deprivation paradigm, and thus the confound of sleep deprivation exists in nearly all of these studies. Reviews of these and other studies of declarative memory enhancement during sleep in humans tend, on the whole, to be skeptical that there is any acceptable evidence at present (e.g. Coolidge, 1974; Siegel, 2001; Vertes and Eastman, 2000; Walker, 2005).

On the other hand, there appears to be mounting evidence for the enhancement of procedural memories in human sleep. Walker (2005) argues that the initial acquisition phase of learning and memory does not appear to rely fundamentally on sleep. This initial stabilization stage (which itself follows acquisition) is characterized by the formation of durable memory representations and resistance to interference, and, like acquisition, develops as time passes. But there is a second stage, consolidation-based enhancement that may show additional learning benefits without further rehearsal. Walker proposes that consolidation-based enhancement may fundamentally rely on several specific sleep stages (but presently only for procedural memories). The specific stages involved may themselves depend on the type of procedural memory, and slow-wave sleep, REM, and stage 2 have all been implicated (Walker, 2005).

Karni *et al.* (1994) first demonstrated consolidation-based enhancement in humans on a procedural visual-spatial discrimination task. Learning was enhanced after a night of sleep but not after 4–12 hours of wakefulness. They also established that selective disruption of REM sleep, but not non-REM, resulted in a loss of these memory gains. Stickgold, James, and Hobson (2000) used the same task as Karni *et al.* and found that the consolidation enhancement was dependent only on the first night of sleep following acquisition. They also found that learning enhancement was correlated with both the amount of slow wave sleep and the amount of REM sleep. Again using the same task, Gais *et al.* (2000) deprived participants of sleep early in the night (presumably of predominately slow-wave sleep) and later in the night (presumably REM and stage 2). They concluded that consolidation-based enhancement might be instigated by slow-wave sleep, whereas REM and stage 2 may solidify and add to the enhancement effect, but that slow-wave sleep was a necessary component. If the latter conclusions are true, then the presently proposed further increases in both slow-wave and REM sleep as a result of the ground sleep transition would have been advantageous for the consolidation-based enhancement of the procedural memories.

In the first of two studies of a procedural motor skills task (sequential finger-tapping), Walker *et al.* (2002) again found consolidation-based enhancement for normal-length periods of sleep immediately following acquisition, or after a period of wakefulness after acquisition then followed by sleep. They found no enhancement effect during a 12-hour awake period following acquisition. When sleep-stage amounts were correlated with enhanced learning, they found that stage 2 amounts were most strongly and positively correlated with learning. In a second study, Walker *et al.* (2003) found that a majority of the consolidation-based enhancement occurred after the first night of sleep following acquisition, but that additional delayed learning did occur on subsequent nights. They also speculated that acquisition learning and delayed learning during sleep were regulated by different mechanisms. Fischer *et al.* (2002) replicated these findings and supported the conclusion that a full night's sleep after acquisition is critical to the delayed enhancement effect. However, they found that learning was positively correlated to REM sleep, but not for stage 2.

In a procedural visuo-motor task, Smith and MacNeill (1994) found that selective deprivation of late night sleep, particularly stage 2, impaired retention. Maquet *et al.* (2003) used a similar task and again demonstrated the sleep-dependent enhancement of memory, and the effect was present after three nights of sleep following acquisition.

Aubrey *et al.* (1999) proposed that the degree of task complexity may be one determining factor in whether slow-wave, REM, or stage 2 sleep are critical to the enhancement of memory. They suggested REM might be more critical to procedural tasks of greater complexity, such as visual discrimination, whereas stage 2 might be more critical to more simple procedural tasks like motor skills. Walker (2005) surmised that if memory enhancement were one of the critical functions of sleep then evolutionarily it would make sense that the different sleep stages were exploited for their differential advantages for various tasks.

Summary

1 Hobson and McCarley proposed an activation-synthesis hypothesis to explain the meaninglessness and randomness of dreaming. They proposed that PGO spikes, arising from the pons, randomly stimulated the areas of the brain resulting in a bizarre array of random visions and thoughts, although often organized into a semi-coherent story. Hobson later retracted his view of the 'meaninglessness' of dreams and saw them as transitory mental illnesses.

2 Winson proposed that REM sleep may have evolved to process and strengthen visuospatial memories critical to survival.

3 I have proposed that sleep, including slow-wave, REM, and dreaming may have evolved for at least three overlapping, non-mutually exclusive reasons: recuperative (protective), adaptive (priming and creativity), and mnemonitive.

CHAPTER 5

Freudian dream interpretation

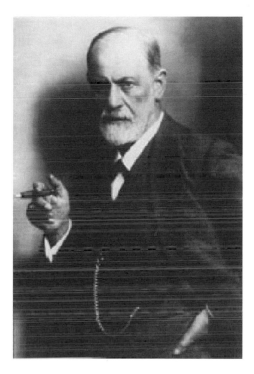

Figure 5.1: Sigmund Freud

Upon my first visit to the British Museum in London, I walked into the majestic round Reading Room, where so many famous scholars have studied. One glass case caught my attention in particular. The British Reading Room staff had encased three first edition books that, in their opinion, had influenced modern thought more than any other works in the past 150 years. Those books were: Charles Darwin's *Origin of Species*, Karl Marx's *Das Kapital*, and Sigmund Freud's *The Interpretation of Dreams*. Being a psychologist myself, I was impressed with the latter choice. Having taught Freud for years, I knew that *The Interpretation of Dreams* did far more than provide Freud's advice on interpreting dreams. In the book, Freud outlined his theory of psychoanalysis, the structure and formation of the psyche, and his guidelines for conducting psychoanalysis, in addition to his theories of dreaming. Also, having read *The Interpretation of Dreams* many times, I knew the book to be an excellent introduction to Freudian theory, with the exception of some of his later works that modified some of his concepts. I also knew, however, that *The Interpretation of Dreams* went far beyond any previous dream work, in that Freud couched dream analysis not only in an elaborate psychotherapeutic technique (psychoanalysis) but also in an elaborate theory of behavior (psychodynamic theory).

Freud was born in 1856 in Freiberg, Austria (now Příbor, Czech Republic) and died of cancer in London in 1939. He considered himself an outsider nearly all his career. First, he grew up Jewish in a Catholic country, and, from early in his academic beginnings, he experienced the vicissitudes of anti-Semitism. Ironically, however, he was an avowed atheist and referred to himself as a 'godless Jew.' In 1877 he studied with Ernst Brücke, a German physiologist, whom Freud saw as the most important teacher in his life, and Freud eventually received his MD degree in 1881. In 1884 he published a paper on the uses of cocaine, particularly its use as an anesthetic for minor eye operations and as a means of relieving depression and morphine addiction. However, in his enthusiasm he overlooked its addictive qualities and became addicted himself for many years. When a close friend died from the addiction, Freud renounced cocaine use and often endured his later cancer operations with only a local anesthetic. In 1885 he received a small grant to study with Jean-Martin Charcot, a French neurologist, who was interested in hysteria and the use of hypnosis to treat it. On November 4, 1899 Freud published his monumental work, *The Interpretation of Dreams*, but it carried the more auspicious publication date of 1900. In 1906 Carl Jung and Freud began the correspondence that would have them visit Clarke University together in 1909, as Freud steadily became world-famous. Despite being chosen as Freud's 'crown prince' of psychoanalysis ('the talking cure'), the theoretical rift between Jung and Freud widened, and they had stopped all correspondence by 1912. In 1923 Freud had the first of many operations on his jaw for the cancer that would eventually kill him 16 years later. In 1927 Freud published *The Future of an Illusion* where he firmly stated his objections to the false illusions of religion and proposed that the human race's only savior was scientific reasoning. In 1929 he continued with his psychoanalysis of culture, and published *Civilization and its Discontents*. In 1933 Freud's writings were publicly burned in Germany under the new Nazi regime. In 1938 the Nazis marched into Austria to cheering throngs. Freud and his family left for Paris and then London. However, one condition for leaving stipulated by the Nazis was that Freud sign an indemnification letter. Freud included the following brazen sentence: 'I can heartily recommend the Gestapo to anyone.' His cancer was finally inoperable, and Freud asked his physician for a series of morphine injections. He died later that night at 3 a.m., on September 23, 1939.

The manifest and latent meaning of dreams

Sigmund Freud advanced in *The Interpretation of Dreams* the hypothesis that dreams had both an obvious or *manifest meaning* and a symbolic or *latent meaning*. The manifest meaning of a dream is simply what appears most obvious as a dream's theme. Freud also used the phrase 'pictorial value' to describe the manifest content of dreams. For example, a college football player told me the following dream:

> I was coming out of the dorm, and people were just standing around. I started to run into them, knocking into them and knocking them over. Just then an airplane swooped over our heads and started machine-gunning them. I wasn't hit.

I think that the obvious or manifest meaning of this dream is easy to interpret. It contains a common theme of hostility or aggression. To come to the conclusion that a 19-year-old football player's dreams contain hostility is not exceptionally helpful. It could be helpful, of course, but Freud and other dream theorists have made the argument that the latent meanings of dreams are far more useful. Freud thought that the latent and symbolic meanings of dreams provided for a much richer interpretation.

Freud thought that the manifest meanings of dreams were chosen from our waking daily life. Much of this material might be from the previous waking day, yet frequently there might also be scenes from our childhood. However, Freud believed that no recent waking idea or scene from the past was chosen randomly. He believed that strong unconscious issues were ultimately selected from the myriad waking ideas and old memories. He thought these unconscious issues were still too scary and powerful to be perceived even by the consciousness of the dream state. Thus, the issues became symbolized or hidden by an automatic process of the psyche. For example, I recently had the following dream:

> I was outside a metal building whose inside consisted of ugly metal beams. I was remembering in the dream that this building had something to do with the draft and that I had been there 30 years ago. A bad feeling welled up inside as I recalled the memory of having been sent a letter to report for my draft physical during the Vietnam War. I tried to remember whom I was with when I was in this building, and I recalled it was two buddies from high school. I remembered their names in my dream. I kept thinking, once one was inside the building, it was too late to resist. We were herded like cattle through various stations until we came out, and then no resistance was possible. But now the building was unused and just a smelly relic. I stood outside in the sunshine and kept thinking, 30 years ago, the draft was like a holocaust for 18-year-olds.

I do not think it is likely that I could pick out my own latent issues in this dream. I could probably figure out something, but I think my own unconscious resistance will prevent me from determining major unconscious themes. However, I present the dream to show how manifest content is not chosen randomly. This dream, whose manifest content was full of anxious themes, appears to remind me of the long-forgotten fears I had of being drafted and sent to Vietnam. Also, it now reminds me of the helplessness I felt. I was only in my second year of college. I wanted to finish my degree. I did not want to be separated from my wife and son, and I did not want to die.

No doubt the themes of helplessness and death are common major issues for nearly everyone and are probably unresolvable. No rationalization is ever fully successful in keeping them at bay, and probably some ego defenses are more successful than others in keeping one's major unconscious issues hidden. However, eventually something in our current daily lives will subtly or unconsciously remind us of our major issues, and invariably we dream about them.

Freud believed that there were at least two major processes operating to turn unconscious issues into manifest content – *condensation* and *displacement*. The process of condensation involves taking more than one unconscious issue and combining them into a single dream image. Freud also called these unconscious issues dream-thoughts and that we should distinguish these from what we actually 'see' in the dreams. What we see, he called dream-elements or dream-content. Thus, there can be more than one correct interpretation, and thus more than one meaning of a single dream element, so Freud said that a dream will be made in the following manner:

> A dream is constructed, rather, by the whole mass of dream-thoughts being submitted to a sort of manipulative process in which those elements which have the most numerous and strongest supports acquire the right of entry into dream-content...the elements of the dream are constructed out of the whole mass of dream-thoughts and each one of those elements is shown to have been determined many times over in relation to the dream-thoughts.

Displacement is a process of transformation where the fearful unconscious issues become changed into approachable subject matter. Freud described the process in the following manner:

> It thus seems plausible to suppose that in the dream-work a psychical force is operating which on the one hand strips the elements which have a high psychical value of their intensity, and on the other hand, by means of overdetermination, creates from elements of low psychical value, new values, which afterwards find their way into the dream-content. If that is so, a trans-ference and displacement of psychical intensities occurs in the process of dream-formation, and it is as a result of these that the difference between the text of the dream-content and that of the dream-thoughts comes about. The process which we are here presuming is nothing less than the essential portion

of the dream-work; and it deserves to be described as 'dream-displacement.' Dream displacement and dream-condensation are the two governing factors to whose activity we may in essence ascribe the form assumed by dreams.

The psychotherapist could use both the manifest and latent content of the dream for discussion in psychotherapy. As I stated earlier, I believe that the manifest content is relatively easy to recognize. For example, in my previously related dream, the overt theme appeared to be anxiety. If we depart from Freudian theory briefly, there is some empirical support that suggests that recent waking anxieties create anxiety dreams. Thus, a therapist might say: 'Fred, your dream contains some obviously anxious themes. What do these anxious feelings make you think about in your current life?' Here, the therapist will simply use a process of free association to find some current worrisome material in Fred's life. However, remember that I stated that manifest content is not that exciting or compelling? I believe that the therapist could possibly help the patient solve their current worry only to find that a plethora of daily worries hurry to replace that solved one. I think that the therapist will benefit the patient more if the therapist can help the patient solve or even begin to think about the 'original' anxiety or even one of them. I believe, like Freud, that it is the early childhood or adolescent issue that triggers the current adult situational anxiety. Because most therapies operate on the principle that awareness, per se, is curative, just having the patient becoming aware that the current anxiety may take the form of an early childhood issue may be helpful, and the therapist does not have to take the responsibility for solving the issue. I trust, like Carl Rogers, a humanistic therapist, that the patient knows best how to solve the problem. If the therapist helps the patient to become aware of the old issue and provides an unconditionally positive or safe psychotherapeutic environment, the patient will eventually provide a correct solution.

Dreams as wish-fulfillment

Freud (1900) stated firmly:

> A dream remains the fulfillment of a wish, no matter in what way the expression of that wish-fulfillment is determined by the currently active material.
> ...[T]he meaning of *every* dream is the fulfillment of a wish, that is to say that there cannot be any dreams but wishful dreams...
> (p. 312)

If we dream of something pleasant, it is easy to think that Freud was right about this dream principle. I have dreamt about old girlfriends, no doubt with a wish to revisit them. I once dreamt about meeting the actress Winona Ryder. Once again, however, these are overt themes. We should get to the latent meanings so as to help our patients more in the long run than the short; so where are the latent meanings in wish-fulfilling dreams? Freud said that it was with dreams about the death of a loved one that his readers presented him with the most arguments about this principle. Yet he stuck to his premise. Yes, even the death of a loved one is a wish-fulfilling dream.

In the simplest (and saddest) of circumstances, we could imagine a loved one in great pain with a terminal illness. We might dream that our loved one dies to remove them from pain or to send them to heaven (or whatever our beliefs might be about an afterlife). Thus, our dream is a wish-fulfilling dream in order to provide a greater good. However, there might also be a lesser good, and that is that we are also removed from a painful situation by their death. No more tears, no more sad times for us, perhaps no more financial burden of the loved one. Perhaps there could even be insurance money? Although our conscious mind may be repelled by the thought, our unconscious mind may not, and it may be useful for our patient's conscious mind to accept this possibility. Excessively strong conscious resistance may suggest excessively strong unconscious desires, and the result could be even more vivid dreams, or much worse. The patient may be involved in an 'accident' with their loved one in real life, and this accident might have been prevented had the therapist been able to confront the patient with their unconscious but frightening desires.

How did Freud explain the death of a loved one who was healthy? At this point, Freud reverted to the heart of his psychoanalytic theory. He offered empirical evidence during his time that males more often dreamt about the death of their fathers and girls about the death of their mothers. Thus, a male who dreams about the death of his father is once again replaying his Oedipus conflict from when he was young and viewed his father as his rival for his mother's affection. Thus, he wished his father out of the picture or dead.

Freud also believed that many feelings, even love, contain an essential ambivalence, so even love has its dark side – hate. Again, our conscious minds may rebel at the thought. 'It is not possible,' a patient says, 'I love my mother; I do not hate her.' However repugnant the thought may be, there must be ways in which the patient's mother had in some way neglected or disappointed the patient. Maybe the patient's mother was too self-absorbed, doted on another sibling, or was not rich enough. Perhaps the patient's mother did not love the patient enough. Perhaps, there were too many other siblings. Perhaps there was a sickly sibling who received most of the mother's attention. It is easy to imagine a patient who feels that their psychological problems are largely due to their mother. According to Freud, there had to be some long-forgotten resentment. It would be impossible for our mothers to have been perfect. Now, perhaps, more than one ancient unconscious issue transforms itself into a wish-fulfilling dream – a loved one's death.

How did Freud explain the dream of the death of a sibling as wish-fulfilling?

For some patients' dreams, this is easy. We do not even have to use Freudian theory. Some patients are on terrible terms with a sibling. The dream death of a sibling may not only represent an unconscious wish but a very conscious wish as well. The history of the world is certainly replete with real examples of fratricide and sororicide, but if we do revert to Freudian theory, he claimed that older and more powerful siblings typically bullied the younger, less powerful ones. The younger siblings had to endure this bullying. However, later in life, they dream of their older sibling's death. According to Freud, it is this old unconscious death wish that has come back, and, somewhat ironically, the dreamer feels guilty about having this dream. The dreamer may even protest to the therapist: 'But I don't wish my brother dead!' According to Freud, the dreamer at one time did wish his brother's death. Also, according to Freud, the manifest content of a dream may be triggered by more than one unconscious element, so dreaming of a brother's death may be the condensation of more than one unconscious issue. However, do not despair that you may not be able to figure out all of the unconscious issues for a dream. Freud also noted that it is in fact never possible to be sure that a dream has been interpreted completely.

Freud's recurring dreams: Otto and Irma

I will use one of Freud's own dreams to highlight this wish-fulfillment principle and to reinforce some of the other points that I have made. In *The Interpretation of Dreams,* Freud presents a dream about his family doctor, Otto:

> My friend Otto was looking ill. His face was brown and he had protruding eyes (p. 303).

Freud offers his own interpretation. He suggests that Otto actually represents Professor R. whom Freud admires, because Professor R. only earned that title later in life, something Freud admitted that he wished very much he could also do (Freud was denied an academic position because of anti-Semitism). So, Freud's interpretation was that he wanted to be a professor.

I could not argue with Freud on this interpretation, because it seems quite plausible. However, remember that manifest content can have more than one unconscious cause, and I strongly believe that we have tremendously strong defenses against the unconscious issues we fear the most. In Freud's case, he actually tells us the issue that he fears the most. After presenting the dream, he says: 'But where was its wish-fulfillment to be found? *Not in avenging myself on my friend Otto...*' (p. 304) [italics mine].

However, Freud appears to have engaged in the ego defense of reaction formation, perhaps, by protesting too much. In one of my most vivid examples of a therapist's naïveté in this regard, one of my master's students had a practicum at the local mental health center. As we began to discuss the case, I asked him why his patient had come to the center. 'Not because she was afraid!' was his strongly stated answer. I asked him why he said that. He said that he asked her that question at the beginning of the interview, and he said that she stated her answer very firmly, 'Not because I'm afraid!' Why did his patient come into the center? Because she was afraid or highly ambivalent about something in her life.

Freud was, at the very least, ambivalent about his feelings for Otto. Certainly, he had consciously positive feelings about Otto. He stated that, 'Otto is my family doctor, and I owe him more than I can ever hope to repay: he has watched over my children's health for many years...' Yet, could it not be that Freud was professionally jealous of Otto? Otto treated Freud's children successfully for years. Couldn't Freud have developed some unconscious resentment towards Otto? After all, Freud was also a physician, but he was prevented from treating his own family members by medical ethics, and Freud gives us a hint of this resentment when he stated earlier in *The Interpretation of Dreams*, '...how awkward it is, when all is said and done, for a physician to ask medical treatment for himself from his professional colleagues.'

Furthermore, was Freud a complete saint? Was he above marital jealousy? Freud wrote that Otto had visited his home on the dream-day and stated, 'my wife remarked that he looked tired and strained.' I could imagine a jealous husband resenting the fact that his wife worried more about his colleague than about him. Freud had also noted, 'I owe him more than I can ever hope to repay...' Therefore, it is not hard to imagine that Freud wished to sicken Otto in his dreams. This way, Otto might die (a slow death!), and Freud would not have to repay the debt. Plus, Freud rids himself of a rival for his children's and wife's affection and rids himself of a professional rival.

If Freud was alive and in dream therapy with me, I might circumvent his resistance by saying: 'You said you did not wish to avenge yourself on your friend Otto. Humor me for a while, and tell me in what possible ways, no matter how remotely possible they may be, that you do wish to avenge yourself upon Otto.' It helps, of course, if the therapist already has some hypotheses about the nature of this unconscious wish. Listening carefully to the patient's life story will help promote this hypothesis formation. Remember, a bad hypothesis is better than no hypothesis (and a good hypothesis is better than a bad one!). You can later test your hypotheses simply by asking your patient questions.

Freud reported many of his own dreams and offered his interpretations. In virtually all of them, there are rich and alternate wish-fulfillment interpretations that Freud does not offer nor could we realistically expect him to. Again, what is hidden wishes to remain so, and no mere superficial probing of the unconscious by the conscious will bring up this material. Here's another example of wish-fulfillment in one of Freud's dreams from *The Interpretation of Dreams*. Irma, he writes, was a young lady who had been one of his patients in psychoanalytic treatment. He said that she was on 'very friendly terms with me and my family.' However, Freud said that her treatment had ended in only partial success, and:

I had proposed a solution to the patient which she seemed unwilling to accept. While we were thus at variance, we had broken off the treatment for the summer vacation. One day I had a visit from a junior colleague, one of my oldest friends [Otto], who had been staying with my patient, Irma, and her family at their country resort. I asked him how he had found her and he answered: 'She's better, but not quite well.' I was conscious that my friend Otto's words, or the tone in which he spoke them, annoyed me. I fancied I detected a reproof in them...
(p. 138)

Freud said he wrote out Irma's case history that night, and the next morning he reported this dream (which I have edited for the sake of brevity):

A large hall – numerous guests, whom we were receiving. Among them was Irma. I at once took her on one side, as though to answer her letter and to reproach her for not having accepted my 'solution' yet. [...] I took her to the window to look down her throat, and she showed no sign of recalcitrance [...] My friend Otto was now standing beside her as well, and my friend Leopold was percussing her through her bodice and saying: 'She has a dull area low down on the left.' [...] My friend Otto had given her an injection...Injections of that sort ought not to be made so thoughtlessly. [...] And probably the syringe had not been clean.
(p.139)

Freud proceeded to analyze this dream, nearly line by line. It consisted of his various associations to the numerous dream elements. He finally summarizes the meaning of the dream as a wish-fulfillment dream whereby he acquits himself of any responsibility for Irma's continuing problems. Furthermore, Freud sees that he tries to blame Otto for Irma's pains, and thus extracts a measure of revenge upon Otto for his imagined reproof of Freud the previous day.

It was a noble attempt by Freud to interpret the latent meanings of his dream. However, given that Freud attached the greatest significance to human sexuality as the origin for psychological problems, it is curious that his interpretation barely addressed this issue, at least with regard to himself. First of all, Freud dreamt of Irma. With his own dream principle, he states that every dream is a dream of wish-fulfillment. Therefore, even the manifest meaning of this dream tells us that he wishes to dream of Irma. After he gives his long interpretation of the meaning of the dream, he tells us she is a young widow, and he brings this fact up right after he states the premier importance of sexuality to nervous disorders like Irma's. Second, Freud introduces Otto into the dream, the same Otto who served as Freud's family physician and his rival. Freud's own interpretation of Otto in the dream is that Freud wishes to blame Otto for Irma's continuing problems, thus absolving himself. Curiously, however, Freud has his friend Leopold, another physician, with Otto standing by, 'percussing' Irma through her bodice. Percussing is a medical procedure whereby the physician strikes or taps the patient's body for diagnostic purposes, and Freud's own interpretation is that good physicians may examine children without their clothes on, but that it is only appropriate to examine adult females with their clothes on. It is, at the very least, an interesting choice of body areas for Freud to have 'wished' his friends to examine. Third, Freud finally has Otto 'inject' Irma, and then worries about a dirty 'syringe.' It appears to me that these images can be viewed as thinly veiled sexual innuendoes. The injection may refer to sexual intercourse, and the dirty syringe might be a syphilitic penis. Before you might object, Freud later stated in *The Interpretation of Dreams*:

> It is fair to say that there is no group of ideas that is incapable of representing sexual facts and wishes.
> (p. 266)

Freud also said in his book that he discussed the problem of prostitution with the governess of his children 'in order to influence her emotional life – for this had not developed quite normally...' and then he dreamt about a word that made him freely associate to the word syphilis.

It is not unreasonable to assume that Freud had repressed sexual desires for Irma. The manifest content of the dream flirts seductively with sexual topics and so does the latent content. Again, if Freud were in therapy with me, and I encountered strong conscious resistance to this interpretation, I might ask Freud to humor me again, and tell me in what ways he might find Irma sexually attractive. On the one hand, I might be accused of encouraging Freud's sexual fantasies. However, becoming aware of sexual desires is different than acting upon them. If one is aware of one's sexual attraction to another, then one has the option of making fully conscious decisions about marital fidelity instead of acting impulsively, and perhaps regretfully, and then claiming that one's infidelity was an 'accident' or making an excuse such as 'I don't know what happened.' This technique does encourage people to take full responsibility for their actions.

Another puzzle for Freud from his critics was the dream of being punished or dreams full of anxiety. How could those possibly be wish-fulfilling dreams? One possibility that Freud suggested was that the ego, although asleep, played a larger role than previously thought in the dream process. Thus, when a repressed desire or wish was expressed in the dream material, the conscious ego reacted indignantly or violently. Thus, the dreamer might be awakened by a sudden burst of anxiety created by the ego or the sleeping dreamer is punished by the ego in the manifest content of the dream for expressing such a disgusting and inappropriate desire. The other possibility offered by Freud is subtly different. Freud thought that the punishment was created by the unconscious, and thus the repressed wish or desire was to be punished. It is fairly easy to imagine the latter could be true for many types of psychopathological disorders, such as the self-defeating personality, or in masochistic personalities. To remain in a true Freudian vein, themes of bondage and punishment are common in surveys of normal, healthy adults. It is not so outlandish then to imagine punishment in dreams as either a repressed desire or a conscious desire.

Freud modifies his stand that all dreams are wish-fulfilling dreams

Nightmares and troubled dreams after traumatic events like war and childhood sexual trauma eventually forced Freud to rethink his adamant stand that all dreams were wish-fulfilling. In his 1920 book, *Beyond the Pleasure Principle*, Freud (1920/1990) reluctantly recognized that nightmares often developed after these traumatic experiences. We will more fully discuss the reasons for his change of heart in Chapter 8, which deals with troubled sleep and dreams. At this point, it may suffice to say that he did modify his stand and came to admit that not all dreams were wish-fulfilling.

Freud's explanation for flying dreams and a physiological explanation

In order to explain flying dreams, Freud reverted to one of his original explanations for many wish-fulfilling dreams. He thought that few children did not have a father or uncle who would throw the child happily into the air (and catch them on the way down). Thus flying dreams, according to Freud, were a desire to be young again, to regress to a happier, more carefree state where most of our primary needs were met without effort. Whether our childhoods were actually happier and more carefree may be irrelevant. For Freud it was enough that we now think that our childhoods were happier and carefree in order to have this wish-fulfilling dream.

There is also a physiological explanation for flying dreams. One interesting phenomenon during REM sleep is *REM incorporation*. One theory has it that, during REM, we may be both paradoxically involved in our dream state and yet semi-aware of our environment. Parents, in particular, may awaken quickly if their children call their name or if a loved one shouts fire. There may be semi-conscious sleep filters that do allow certain material into our sleep consciousness to awaken us. Also, some physiological urges obviously make their way into our dream material. The most common of these urges is the desire to urinate, and frequently in the early morning when our bladders are reaching their fullest limits, our dream story may turn into a search for a toilet.

When I was growing up in Miami, we used to fly model planes with tiny gas engines. One morning, I dreamt I was flying my favorite model plane (a P-40

Warhawk), when I pictured it getting closer and closer to flying over my head. In reality, outside, a Flying Boxcar (C-119) was spraying our neighborhood for a fruit fly infestation. As the plane outside flew right over our house, the plane in my dream flew right over my head, and the noise outside became the noise inside, and I nearly fell out of my bed, I was awakened so abruptly. This is an example of REM incorporation, where REM sleep selectively incorporates environmental and internal physiological stimuli into our dreams.

Thus, flying dreams may actually be examples of REM incorporation of a physiological stimulus. This stimulus may be the phenomenon of muscle atony that occurs at the onset of REM sleep. In fact, before the discovery in 1953 that vivid dream sleep was accompanied by rapid eye movements, the onset of dream sleep was measured by a sudden loss of muscle tone in the neck muscles. The choice of neck muscles was merely convenient, because the other EEG electrodes were already pasted about the head. Thus, the overall sudden loss of muscle tone at the onset of REM sleep may have been incorporated into the dream as flying, soaring, or being cast into the air like a child. We might also explain the frequent dream of being awake and paralyzed as a variant of the same REM incorporation phenomenon. The dreamer is not awake but dreams that they are, and, further, the dreamer incorporates the loss of muscle tone as being awake but paralyzed.

A REM sleep explanation for reports of alien abductions

It is also possible that REM incorporation of muscle atony may also explain the reports of alien abductions. Many seemingly normal people (other than their belief in UFOs) have reported being abducted by aliens. Their reports frequently contain either the story that they are in bed, paralyzed, or being examined by the aliens, or they have been abducted aboard a spaceship, are paralyzed or bound in some way, and are being examined by the aliens. It is possible that these people are simply fulfilling a wish by dreaming about aliens (which is their conscious belief), and at the same time, their sleep filters are trying to explain the muscle atony accompanying REM sleep. Thus, they dream they are paralyzed or bound. Also, this may account for why their reports seem so real and by any of the standard physiological measures of lying (like galvanic skin response), there is no indication that they are making up their stories. Certainly, their stories seem real! For certain, their stories are no less real than a vivid dream or nightmare, particularly the emotion or affect that is generated during the dream. We might argue with these reports and say, 'but it was only a dream,' but we should be careful about denying the strength of the emotion or affect. How silly we would be if we said, 'but it was not real anxiety,' or 'it was not real fear.'

Summary

1 Freud believed in the manifest or obvious meaning of dreams and in the latent, hidden, or symbolic meaning of dreams. He thought the latter might be more useful to interpret.

2 Freud believed in dream condensation, where more than one unconscious issue could condense into a single dream image.

3 Freud believed in dream displacement, where fearful or highly charged unconscious issues could be changed into a more approachable subject matter.

4 Freud initially believed that all dreams are wish-fulfilling dreams but later admitted some kinds of nightmares, especially after highly traumatic events, may not be wish-fulfilling.

5 Freud believed that any dream idea could represent sexual facts and wishes.

6 Aspects of our current external environment may be directly incorporated into our dreams. Physiological states (such as a full bladder) can also be immediately incorporated into our dreams.

7 Flying dreams may be examples of REM incorporation of the muscle atony that occurs at the onset of REM sleep.

8 Reports of alien abductions and muscle paralysis may actually be wish-fulfilling REM dreams accompanied by muscle atony.

CHAPTER 6

Jungian dream interpretation

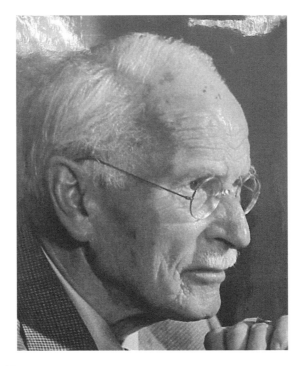

Figure 6.1: Carl Jung

Carl Jung (1875–1961) was a Swiss psychiatrist and contemporary of Freud, although 19 years his junior. He began studying with Freud in 1907. Their relationship developed to the point where Freud chose Jung to carry on his psychoanalytic activities, and called Jung his 'son' and 'crown prince.' However, Jung was obviously independently brilliant and creative, and ultimately developed a more positive view of the unconscious. They also disagreed on the nature of God. Freud maintained that God did not exist and was created out of reaction formation. Jung saw the development of God images in all cultures as a kind of proof of God's existence. By 1914, their split was so divisive that, although Freud lived 25 more years, they never spoke to one another again.

Jung's written works were always designed for sophisticated audiences. Less than two years before his death, he was approached by the British Broadcasting Corporation for an in-depth interview. The program was seen by a book publisher who thought it a shame that Jung, intensely fascinating, humorous, and charming, had never been popular with the masses. Jung's writings were considered too difficult to understand for the average reader. The book publisher approached the TV interviewer about having Jung write a book for the average person. The TV interviewer thought it was a great idea and approached Jung. Jung listened to a two-hour presentation while in his garden and then firmly said no.

The TV interview had reached people with whom Jung would not normally have come into contact, and he was quickly inundated with letters from all over the world. However, that alone did not change his mind. He went to sleep one night and had a dream. In the dream, instead of his customary sophisticated audience, he saw himself in a public place addressing a huge throng of people. They were not only listening to him carefully, but they also understood him! Because Jung's psychological theories were intimately tied to dream messages, he could hardly refuse to listen to this prophetic dream. A short while later, he agreed to do the book, called *Man and His Symbols*. The book had two conditions attached to its undertaking: it was to be a collective effort by Jung and his closest colleagues; and the TV interviewer would serve as the arbiter between the authors and the publishers. Jung planned the structure of the book, chose his colleagues and their topics, and wrote the main and first chapter, 'Approaching the unconscious.' He died on June 6, 1961, just ten days after he had completed his chapter and had approved the drafts of the other authors.

Although seemingly impossible, Jung probably believed in the power of the interpretation of dreams even more than Freud. I once opened a fortune cookie that read, 'A dream of happiness is real happiness.' In a way, this sums up Jung's philosophy of dreaming: dreams are as real as any other psychological phenomena. Furthermore, dreams are intensely personal. They cannot be decoded by any standard glossary of meanings. Thus, you cannot buy a dream interpretation dictionary, look up dreams about lobsters, and read that it means your father was a callous person. Jung thought that dreams were messages from an individual's unconscious, and, even though all people share a collective unconscious, the messages are, nevertheless, personal and individual. A person's dreams cannot be interpreted by a glossary, codebook, or dictionary. On the importance of dreams and these messages (in an anthology of his writings published in 1970, *Psychological Reflections*), Jung wrote the following:

> The dream is a little hidden door in the innermost and most secret recesses of the soul, opening into that cosmic night which was psyche long before there was any ego-consciousness, and which will remain psyche no matter how far our ego-consciousness extends. (p. 53)
>
> Nobody doubts the importance of conscious experience; why then should we doubt the significance of unconscious happenings? They also are part of our life, and sometimes more truly a part of it for weal or woe than any happenings of the day. (p. 53)

> Dream psychology opens the way to a general comparative psychology from which we may hope to gain the same understanding of the development and structure of the human psyche as comparative anatomy has given us concerning the human body. (p. 54)

Freud vacillated somewhere in between standard meanings and personal meanings for dream symbols. Freud clearly rejected strict decoding methods for interpreting dreams, yet he found fascinating ancient dream interpretation approaches as in the *Oneirocritica*. As noted earlier, the *Oneirocritica* used a combination of both standard meanings and also the circumstances of the dreamer, such as the dreamer's occupation.

Freud also noted that dream symbols are as old as language itself. He wrote:

> Dreams make use of this symbolism for the disguised representation of their latent thoughts. Incidentally, many of the symbols are habitually or almost habitually employed to express the same thing. Nevertheless, the peculiar plasticity of the psychical material [in dreams] must never be forgotten. (Freud, 1900; p. 387)

Only 12 pages after this firm warning, Freud entitles a section in *The Interpretation of Dreams*, The Genitals Represented by Buildings, Stairs and Shafts. Personally, I think Jung's approach to dream symbol interpretation makes more sense. Although the dream of a key going into a lock might be tempting for Freudians to interpret as a sexual act, it seems intuitively more reasonable to vary the interpretation for a prisoner, locksmith, or treasure hunter. In *Man and his Symbols*, Jung wrote:

> It is plain foolishness to believe in ready-made systematic guides to dream interpretation, as if one could simply buy a reference book and look up a particular symbol. No dream symbol can be separated from the individual who dreams it, and there is no definite or straightforward interpretation in any dream. Each individual varies so much in the way that his unconscious complements or compensates his conscious mind that it is impossible to be sure how far dreams and their symbols can be classified at all.
> (Jung, 1968; p. 38)
> It is for this reason that I have always said to my pupils: 'Learn as much as you can about symbolism; then forget it all when you are analyzing a dream.'
> (p. 42)

The compensatory nature of dreams

Jung thought symbols represented more than their obvious meaning, and he thought this wider 'unconscious' meaning could never be fully understood. He traveled throughout the world examining the symbols of various cultures, but he felt that all people produced symbols 'unconsciously and spontaneously' through their dreams. He also viewed consciousness as a recent and slowly developed process, and he thought that dreams were transmissions of unconscious impulses and reactions to consciousness. Freud called them *archaic remnants* that could not be explained by anything currently in the dreamer's life, and he thought they might be the 'aboriginal, innate, and inherited shapes of the human mind.' However, Jung objected to the idea that they were simply remnants. The word 'remnant' has the connotation of a scrap, a leftover, or being unused. Jung thought that these unconscious messages were far more important than that. He felt that dreams served a compensatory function; that is, dream messages were attempts to compensate for 'a particular defect in the dreamer's attitude to life.'

Jung stated two fundamental points of dreams:

First, the dream should be treated as a fact, about which one must make no previous assumption except that it somehow makes sense; and second, the dream is a specific expression of the unconscious.

Jung noted that dreams do have a definite and *purposeful structure* which usually indicated an idea or intention. Jung felt that this purpose was not always understandable but nevertheless very important. Thus he said this about a dreams and its intention:

Its dimensions in time and space are quite different; to understand it you must examine it from every aspect just as you may take an unknown object in your hands and turn it over and over until you are familiar with every detail of its shape.
(Jung, 1970; p. 64)

Jung believed that consciousness had a natural tendency to fear and deny the unknown. This tendency, called *misoneism*, Jung borrowed from anthropologists. It described a fear of new things, a fear of novelty. Thus, Jung was not surprised that people resisted the meanings of their dreams, even when dreams were trying to strike a balance. It was this latter tendency, the compensatory nature of dreams, that Jung felt was so important. However, Jung did not want us to view dreams, necessarily, as friends, or guides, or as moralistic. Dreams simply strike a balance between the 'lopsided nature of ...conscious mind' and the unconscious. Dreams are not moralistic. Jung wrote:

Our actual knowledge of the unconscious shows that it is a natural phenomenon and that, like Nature herself, it is at least *neutral*. It contains all aspects

of human nature – light and dark, beautiful and ugly, good and evil, profound and silly.
(Jung, 1968; p. 94)

One cannot afford to be naïve in dealing with dreams. They originate in a spirit that is not quite human, but is rather a breath of nature – a spirit of the beautiful and generous as well as of the cruel goddess.
(Jung, 1968; p. 36)

About the necessity of the compensatory nature of dreams, Jung wrote:

For the sake of mental stability and even physiological health, the unconscious and the conscious must be integrally connected and thus move on parallel lines. If they are split apart or 'dissociated,' psychological disturbance follows. In this respect, dream symbols are the essential message carriers from the instinctive to the rational parts of the human mind, and their interpretation enriches the poverty of consciousness so that it learns to understand again the forgotten language of the instincts.
(Jung, 1968; p. 37)

One example of this unconscious compensatory nature of dreams I saw in the dream of a 19-year-old college freshman. She was my patient for ten weeks at a campus counseling center. She was an outstanding tennis player, tall, blonde, and buxom. Her presenting problem, she said, was her weight. Although she did not appear overweight by any means, we never missed a session without at least some reference to her 'weight problem.' Then she had this dream:

I had this dream where I went downtown and I wasn't dressed. I was naked, and there were all these people looking at me.

I immediately thought of Freud's wish-fulfillment principle and his interpretation that this dream was an old childhood wish to run about carefree and naked. I gently suggested to her the idea that the dream might contain a secret wish. She almost immediately and cheerfully agreed and suggested that she felt overwhelmed by her first year of college and all the work. She thought that the dream might be telling her that she did wish to be free of her studies and responsibilities, but then I remembered Jung's advice:

...explore the content of the dream with the utmost thoroughness.

and his injunction:

Let's get back to the dream. What does the *dream* say?

I asked her what other kind of message the dream might be sending her. I was also direct. My intuition told me she was secretly proud about something. I remembered Fritz Perl's idea that, behind some secret we are ashamed to tell anyone, there is an aspect of that shame that we are secretly proud of. 'What are you proud of about in this dream?' I asked her. She thought about it only briefly and said, 'My breasts.' It was the first time in therapy that I heard her say anything positive about her body. She then got quiet, and, as if in response to her own thoughts, she said, 'Well, I can't very well go about bragging about them, can I?' We both agreed that she probably could not, but I offered her the explanation that perhaps it was the one-sidedness of her complaints about her body that made her unconsciousness force a compensatory balance. This example also provides support for Freud's idea that a single dream element may have been condensed from more than one dream thought or latent issue.

Jung's patients were frequently in their late thirties to early fifties and economically successful. Just as frequently they often had a similar complaint. Despite their material successes, they were bored. Jung interpreted this boredom as a symptom of the split between the conscious and unconscious parts of the psyche. Boredom was a symptom that this person had cut off their unconscious mind and that this person had ignored the rich symbolic history presented by their dreams. No wonder material successes brought little satisfaction. Their ultimate and most satisfying treasure was within.

However, once again, do not be misled by dreams. For some patients, Jung did not discuss dreams. Remember my master's student who thought his patient had come to him but 'not because she was afraid?' Even in their first session, he was interpreting her dream about her hands on fire, offering her his rich and learned insights from his voracious dream readings. I learned she was unemployed, on welfare, single, and about to lose her two children to social services for neglect. Yet he wanted to talk about her dreams! I was certain that this was a situation where she was already overwhelmed by her unconscious thought processes, and I was correct. My student told me that she believed in dreams, the power of crystals, and followed zodiacal advice like a religion. I explained to my student that this woman was already in contact with her unconscious, in fact, she was overwhelmed by it. In a case like this, Jung might have advised driving a wedge between her unconscious thoughts and impulses, and her flimsy consciousness. Her therapy needed to consist of developing her conscious autonomy in very specific ways, like how to get a job and how to keep her children. Instead of therapy homework like bringing in a dream, she should be thinking of ways to get a job. If that was too difficult, then she might even be asked to bring into therapy the classifieds section of the newspaper, and together she and her therapist might go over the job advertisements. Further therapy might consist of checking bus routes, how to go shopping for food for her children, etc.

Apparently, Jung was a masterful and intuitive therapist, and he realized that one can teach others the knowledge and skills of therapeutic techniques, but there still remained the art of therapy, which could not be taught. When a patient came to Jung complaining of insomnia, Jung sang a lullaby and put his patient to sleep. When a patient said they felt cut off from their religion, Jung asked for a Bible, and they did Bible readings.

Fortunately, however, most good therapists believe that practice, time, and experience does make one a better therapist. There is a popular sports story that a famous sports figure player, after making a great play or sinking a great shot, heard a critic say that he was just lucky. The player is reputed to have said, 'The harder I work, the luckier I get.' I think this practice principle also holds for dream analysis.

Dreams as a spontaneous self-portrayal

As early as more than 2500 years ago, in India's holy book, the Upanishads, came this quote about dreams, 'There are no [real] chariots in that state, no horses, no roads but he himself [creates] chariots, horses, and roads...He indeed is the maker.' Jung continually hammered home this fact. He viewed that dreams may be a reflection of:

> ineluctable truths, philosophical pronouncements, illusions, wild fantasies, memories, plans, anticipations, irrational experiences, even telepathic visions, and heaven knows what besides.
> (Jung, 1970; p. 57)

More importantly, Jung saw them essentially as a spontaneous self-portrayal in a symbolic form. He wrote:

> ...[Dreams] are nothing less than self-portraits of the psychic life-process.
> (Jung, 1970; p. 56)
> The whole dream-work is essentially subjective, and a dream is a theatre in which the dreamer is himself the scene, the player, the prompter, the producer, the author, the public, and the critic.
> (Jung, 1970; p. 66)

I think that there is ample evidence, highly obvious, ancient, and logical, that dreams are an entirely spontaneous self-product. Jung, in particular, thought that every image in a dream potentially contained a useful self-reflection. If you falter or begin to doubt in your examination of any aspect or image in a patient's dream, remember that Jung felt that all of these images might be spokes of a wheel. Ultimately, any of these spokes may lead us to the patient's center. What might be at the center? If we use dreams as our vehicle, then we may come into contact with the most ancient wisdom of our own psyche. Jung envisioned this wisdom as a two-million-year-old person within us. It is the accumulation of two million years of purposeful, intelligent, and wonderfully creative evolution. He wrote:

Together the patient and I address ourselves to the two-million-year-old man that is in all of us. In the last analysis, most of our difficulties come from losing contact with our instincts, with the age-old unforgotten wisdom stored up in us. And where do we make contact with this old man in us? In our dreams. (Jung, 1970; p.76)

The archetypal nature of dreams

Jung believed that the psyche consisted of all of our emotions, thoughts, and behaviors, and had three major parts: the ego, which functions on a conscious level; the personal unconscious, which contains forgotten, suppressed experiences or experiences that fail to attain a conscious level; and the collective unconscious, an inherited part of our psyche whose contents may never have been conscious. This idea of the collective unconscious was one of Jung's most controversial hypotheses and, perhaps, the most fascinating.

The personal unconscious for Jung contained complexes. These are clusters of thoughts, feelings, and memories that may have been conscious at one point, but now have been relegated to the personal unconscious by suppression or repression. Also, in the personal unconscious are fleeting thoughts or feelings that, for a variety of reasons, did not attain consciousness. However, these complexes have ramifications for the ego, because we will avoid, hesitate, or postpone actions that arouse our complexes. All of the latter actions will occur without our conscious awareness of the reasons! Jung once said:

A person does not have a complex; the complex has him.

Although the present day usage of the word 'complex' does originate from Jung, his idea about an inherited unconscious has probably created greater interest. Freud had earlier called the symbolic images in dreams 'archaic remnants.' Jung strongly objected to the notion that dream symbols had any connotation as being 'lifeless' or 'meaningless.' Jung viewed dreams as a kind of bridge between the ancient pictorial and symbolic language of the instinctive world and the conscious rational world. It is important to remember that Jung viewed the unconscious as a repository or museum of human evolutionary history. Jung wrote:

Just as the human body represents a whole museum of organs, each with a long evolutionary history behind it, so we should expect to find that the mind is organized in a similar way. It can no more be a product without history than is the body in which it exists. By 'history' I do not mean the fact that the mind builds itself up by conscious reference to the past through language and other culture traditions. I am referring to the biological, prehistoric, and unconscious development of the mind in archaic man, whose psyche was still close to that of the animal.

This immensely old psyche forms the basis of our mind, just as much as the structure of our body is based on the general anatomical pattern of the mammal. The trained eye of the anatomist or the biologist finds many traces of this original pattern in our bodies. The experienced investigator of the mind can similarly see the analogies between the dream pictures of modern man and the products of the primitive mind, its 'collective images,' and its mythological motifs.
(Jung, 1968; p. 57)

In dreams, Jung believed that symbols occurred spontaneously, and they always stood for something more than the superficial meaning. However, their origins are hidden so deep in our past evolutionary history, that Jung believed they had no human source. At some level, Jung agreed with Freud about their nature: aboriginal, innate, and inherited shapes. Jung called these images 'archetypes' or 'primordial images.' Jung cautioned against interpreting them as the simple equivalent of a mythological image. The actual dream symbol was a conscious representation of the 'ancient, involuntary spontaneous manifestations of the collective unconscious.' It is a collective unconscious, because all humans have universally inherited relatively similar archetypes.

Jung's arguments for these tendencies to form images come from animal instincts. He thought that it was not logical to assume that each newly born human would have to learn every specific way that humans behave. He argued that the 'collective thought patterns of the human mind are innate and inherited.' Could it be, he asked, that only humans are devoid of their evolutionary past in their psyches?

In fact, he argued that the evolutionary development of human consciousness might have been caused by an archetype. He gave the example of a bushman who killed his son out of frustration and anger while fishing, and then remembers this 'moment of pain' forever. Jung thought that this emotional pain had the effect of waking people up and making them pay attention to what they are doing. If this awakening put someone at an adaptive advantage, then that person's genetic information was more likely to get into the gene pool in subsequent generations. In the case of the angry bushman, Jung even felt that there may have been an 'archetype at work for a long time in the unconscious, skillfully arranging circumstances that will lead to a crisis.' Thus, Jung saw archetypes as dynamic factors, making themselves known through impulses. As long as modern people protected themselves from the recognition of these archetypes, Jung thought that they would never be masters of their own souls.

The five major archetypes of the psyche

According to Jung, five of these archetypes have evolved to the point where they exert a greater influence on the psyche. They are (i) animus, the male side of our personality; (ii) anima, a female side to our personality; (iii) persona, the many roles we play for society's sake; (iv) the shadow, a dark, passionate, murderous, yet creative side of our personality; and finally (v) the self, an integrating force that attracts all other archetypes in a holistic, beneficial, unifying way. The archetypes are not inherited as specific ideas or symbols. Jung proposed that they are more like inherited predispositions to think in certain ways or to think about particular cross-cultural and universal themes, like God or mother. They are, as Jung said, 'forms without content.'

In dream interpretation, I have found it useful to examine these archetypes in a patient's dreams. However, I have found it the most useful to concentrate, at least initially, upon animus and anima, and interpret all male and female characters in a dream as the male and female sides of the dreamer's personality. Thus, even though a patient dreams about their mother, I would interpret this character as the mother side of their own personality. However, the five major archetypes do interact with and influence each other continually.

Animus and anima

Jung thought that each of us, regardless of gender, has both male and female psychological and physiological sexual characteristics. Although present research leads us to believe that the single strongest component to our adult sexual identity is inherited (Coolidge, Thede, and Young, 2002), our environment also impacts on the expression of this sexual identity, and our environment obviously contains both male and female influences.

Are there any symbols for the Jungian idea of our inchoate bisexual nature? Indeed, there are. Ometeotl was the first god to exist, according to the Aztecs. Ometeotl means 'two-god,' and Ometeotl was not only self-created but was also male and female. Interestingly, Ometeotl governed heaven at its highest level. This place was called Omeyocan, which means 'place of duality,' and, as a couple, Ometeotl produced four of the Aztecs' great deities. Hermaphroditus of Greek mythology is, of course, a classic archetypal symbol of bisexuality. Hermaphroditus rejected the love of a water nymph, and when he later bathed in her pool she clung so tightly to him that they became one person with a woman's breasts and a man's genitals.

Jung also proposed that the psychological sexual component of masculinity, animus, is typically repressed and unconscious in females, and the psychological sexual component of femininity, anima, is repressed and unconscious in males. There is also an archetypal duality in these gender archetypes, that is, they both have positive and negative attributes. Anima's positive female attributes are characterized by feelings, emotionality, sentimentalism, finding the right inner values, kindness, romance, gentleness, and wisdom. When a man pays attention to his anima, he may express himself creatively through 'writing, painting, sculpture, musical composition, or dancing.' Jung ascribed the common stereotypes in our society for his gender attributes. A very popular positive anima symbol is Mother Nature. We could add Magna Mater (a Roman mother goddess), the Blessed Virgin Mary; Sita, Radha, and Parvati from the Hindu Mahabharata; Aphrodite and Hera from Greek mythology; the Egyptian mother goddess, Neith, goddess Isis and the sky goddess Nut; Nu Gua, creator and protector of humanity from Chinese mythology; Glinda the good witch of the north from the Wizard of Oz; Princess Leia from Star Wars; and Goldberry, Lady Arwen, and Lady Galadriel from the Hobbit Trilogy.

The negative side of anima involves seduction and betrayal, being irrational or illogical, being overcome by emotion, irritability, depressed moods, insecurity, and a plethora of fears. According to Jung, the negative aspects of anima have been symbolized in many cultures by witches, the Germanic singing Lorelei who enticed men to their death, Greek sirens who also sang men to death by hunger, Kali, the murderous side of Parvati with her earrings of corpses, Jezebel and Delilah from the Bible, and the evil Baba Yaga in Russian folklore.

The positive attributes of animus are strength, rationality and logic, action, courage, truthfulness, and 'spiritual profundity.' Its negative attributes are brutality, recklessness, silence, stubbornness, emotional coldness, dogmatism, and inaccessibility. Positive animus can be symbolized by Tarzan, Hemingway, Spock the Vulcan and Captain Kirk from Star Trek, Bilbo, Frodo and Strider from the Hobbit trilogy, Luke Skywalker and Obi Wan Kenobi from Star Wars, Ghandi, Martin Luther King, Jesus, and Buddha.

Jung thought the strength of these attributes in an individual came from our parents; a man receives his individual attributes for better or worse from his mother, and the woman's animus comes from her father. For example, an unloving, uncaring mother may imbue a man's unconscious anima with a mean, 'waspish,' 'poisonous' attitude according to von Franz, a Jungian disciple.

The persona

Animus and anima are also influenced by the persona archetype. The persona is a mask or role that we provide for society's sake. The persona is likely to consist of many different masks, and almost all of them operate totally without our awareness. For example, at home I may play the role of good husband with my wife, stern father with my youngest teenage daughter, professor at the university, and then rock star when I play music in nightclubs. These roles actually help me to be more efficient and thus promote my adaptation and success in my dealings with society, because I do not have to reexamine how I am going to act in every new situation or interaction with others. However, there is a danger in over-identification with one's persona. For example, medical doctors, perhaps involved in daily life-or-death decisions, may over-identify with their doctor's mask of confidence. Many times, they may be quite unsure of the outcome of their decisions in a hospital, but they cannot act as if they are unsure. Acting unsure would upset the patient, the patient's family, and the hospital staff. However, it is possible that some MD's carry this 'act' or persona home where they confidently espouse family advice with the same surety, officiality, and dogmatism. Typically, this style of parenting and spousing does not create happiness or engender love in family members. Politicians may also over-identify with their smiling, glad-handing personas.

Potentially, under-identification with persona is also a problem. Who has rejected personas in our society? Some of my students propose that rebels, like bikers, have rejected society's demands for a persona. However, they are as guilty as professors in creating a persona. On the surface, it is still a persona, a biker's persona but a persona nonetheless. A biker's persona consists of riding a Harley-Davidson motorcycle (never a Honda, even if it looks like a Harley!), wearing black clothes, a black vest, boots, having a chain from one's wallet to a belt or a belt loop, a motorcycle chain for a belt, and perhaps a tattoo of a spiderweb on the elbows. No, a biker's persona may superficially appear to be a rejection of a societal persona, but it is still a persona and a very strong one. Notice, also, that a biker's persona helps a biker to adapt to his or her biker's society. When a biker dressed in their colors pulls up on a Harley to a biker's rally, they 'fit in,' and they are accepted as a member of that society without undue examination or challenge.

Probably a hermit is a good example of someone who has rejected his or her persona. The hermit is a classic loner who resists the masks of society, including son or daughter, brother or sister, friend or enemy. I read a story about a true hermit, a society dropout, who lived deep in a South American jungle. A journalist trudged for days through the jungle and stumbled upon this hermit's hut. The journalist was amazed that a formerly civilized person would live this far from people and so deep in the jungle. The journalist thought, perhaps, that the hermit's tale would make a great story. However, the hermit's first words to the journalist were, 'When are you leaving?'

Our personas, then, usually keep our gender roles tightly defined. Thus, a man's 'manly' persona keeps his anima repressed, and a feminine persona may keep a woman's animus repressed. Jung believed that it was necessary to liberate these repressed aspects of our psyche in order for us to develop to our complete potential. However, it may not be enough to simply liberate a man's anima nor a female's animus. The liberation must be coupled by a reintegration of both gender archetypes, and this is a difficult task. A man may become feminized by allowing his anima to develop, but he must be able to join and synthesize his two gender archetypes so that they exist in harmony and so that his animus is not subjugated in the process. I had a friend who was getting married for the second time. We were all in our 30s and 40s. Six of us got together on the eve of his bachelor party. What should we do? Interestingly, opinion was evenly divided: go out and party, or stay home and talk meaningfully. The groom made his decision that we would stay home and talk. Drink, yes, but talk, and that is what we did for hours. The next day, we were asked by our girlfriends and wives what we did. Ironically, there was some laughter and kidding about what we had chosen. This reflects a man's dilemma: how to develop and release anima without losing animus.

A woman's dilemma, of course, is equally complex. For example, the emphasis on women's sports has been a tremendous boon to their psychical development. It has developed confidence, camaraderie, healthy competition, courage, physical development, and many other positive attributes, and this experience was virtually unavailable to women only 25 years ago. However, it has not been without a cost. Women who participate in sports have been criticized by their own mothers, brother, fathers, boyfriends, and even by some other women as being too masculine, too physical, etc. A woman can also over-embrace this developing animus in the form of athleticism and as a consequence ridicule her brother (who is releasing his anima) for staying home and painting. The dilemma for the woman is how to express her animus yet keep her anima, being able to release animus but being able to integrate those aspects with her anima. The traditional old guards in every society are slow to relinquish their control and suppression. They (sometimes religious leaders, sometimes politicians, etc.) typically fear change (Jung's term was misoneism) and protect the traditional animus in males and anima in females.

The shadow

Another major archetype is the *shadow*. The shadow is the dark side of our personality. It is everything we refuse to admit about ourselves, and thus it visits us in our dreams, usually symbolized in the forms of people we hate. As von Franz (a close colleague of Jung) wrote (in *Man and his Symbols*):

> When an individual makes an attempt to see his shadow, he becomes aware of (and often ashamed of) those qualities and impulses he denies in himself but can plainly see in other people – such things as egotism, mental laziness, and sloppiness; unreal fantasies, schemes, and plots; carelessness and cowardice; inordinate love of money and possessions ...
> (Jung, 1968; p. 174)

The shadow houses our ancient animal instincts. It is the source of our strongest emotions, creativity, vigor, and spontaneity. However, it is the shadow in us that allows us to kill other people, to be mean, spiteful, and hateful. Once the shadow has been aroused to action, particularly rage and anger, there is no reasoning with it. If the shadow and the conscious forces of the ego act in unity, the great forces of the shadow can translate into good works, prodigious tasks, and the like. However, if the shadow cannot sublimate its energies, then a person may self-destruct or harm others. Because the shadow is also a museum for our ancient primitive instincts, Jung postulated that it also contained the adaptive ability to make quick and proper decisions without undue hesitation. Again, however, if a person has worked to understand, release, and integrate their shadow, then their quick decisions may be effective and beneficial. If the shadow has been repressed or acts unbridled, the results may be highly ineffective or detrimental. Furthermore, inevitable conflict results when we project our shadow onto others. Von Franz saw political agitations as created by the projection of our shadows. She saw the projection of the shadow as 'obscuring our view of our fellow men, spoiling objectivity, and thus spoiling all possibility of genuine human relationships.' She also noticed the Herculean task of trying to understand the shadow, because it is sometimes experienced as an irresistible impulse, and it resists being known or bridled. Simply trying to be honest with oneself does not often succeed. She noted that it might take a 'brick...to drop on one's head to put a stop to shadow drives and impulses.' Sometimes, she noted, a monumental 'heroic decision' may stop the destruction from the shadow, but it is not likely. As an example of this brick-to-the-head phenomenon, I had a talented musician friend with a shadowy dark side: illegal drug use. He was finally arrested for only the first time after 12 years of various illegal drug use. However, it was a minor charge, and was likely to be dismissed in court. While waiting to go to trial and swearing to me he was finished with drugs, he bought an illegal drug that was badly synthesized. He had a psychotic reaction, and he tried to remove his fingernails with a knife. He ended up in an emergency room nearly bleeding to death and in the throes of a psychotic episode that lasted for hours. Apparently and hopefully, that was his brick to the head. It may have stopped his self-destructive drug use. It may have bridled his shadow while he seeks healthier releases for it.

The shadow has been symbolized by dark destructive forces for time immemorial. One of the oldest symbols of the shadow comes from the ancient Persian religion, Zoroastrianism. Their essential tenet was a dualistic struggle between a god of good, Ormuzd, and the spirit of evil and darkness, Ahriman. Zoroastrianism also had a prescription for living one's life that consisted of a trinity: good thoughts, good words, and good deeds. Thus, Ahriman is probably one of the earliest symbols of the shadow. The Christian Bible has Satan, the Hindu Ramayana has Ravana who kidnapped Sita, and the Hindu trinity has the Shiva, the destroyer.

Like the other archetypes, the shadow also contains a duality of evil and good. One good aspect of the shadow, as previously mentioned, is its ability to make quick decisions. The shadow is also seen in the creative process. Interestingly, extremely creative artists like Picasso, Dali, and Jackson Pollack had a destructive element in their creativity. They were able to translate into their pictures and sculptures their inner realities, and these realities were personal, highly original, and destructive in the sense that they copied no other artists. They were able to explicate their inner forces in such a way that other people were able to recognize and appreciate the unconscious representations, although perhaps not fully understanding what they saw. Some people gave their art the highest of compliments in the world of symbols by saying, 'I don't know what it means, but I like it.'

The self archetype and individuation

The last of the major archetypes is the *self*, and it was considered the most important by Jung. The self archetype attracts all the other archetypes. It is a unifying force in the psyche. It is a self-actualizing force. It motivates a person to become whole. Jung's favorite symbol of the self was a *mandala,* which is a Sanskrit word for circle. Mandalas are frequently seen in ancient eastern and oriental art, particularly in religious works. They usually consist of circles within an outer square and squares within the inner circles. Jung thought the circles represented wholeness or oneness, and the squares represented another ancient numerical archetype of fourness or *quarternity*. Fourness has been symbolized, according to Jung, by our representation of the seasons into winter, spring, summer, and fall, the ancient elements of earth, wind, fire, and water, the four horsemen of the apocalypse, etc. Again, the unconscious influence of the self archetype and the quarternity archetype can be seen in modern culture as well. In the Wizard of Oz, Dorothy's search to get 'home' may reflect an active, conscious attempt to understand her unconscious self and to sense a 'oneness' and 'wholeness' in doing so. There is a classic quarternity in her search, the Scarecrow, the Tinman, the Cowardly Lion, and, of course, the leader of her search, Dorothy herself. When Glinda told her the secret of returning 'home,' it seemed all too easy and simple. Remember, Dorothy was told that she herself contained the secret to getting home. It was not in Oz, the dazzling external world. It was not through a Wizard (no matter how wonderful a wizard he was), although the Wizard may have symbolized both the positive animus and the self archetypes. Dorothy herself was the answer. Jung viewed this process as an assimilation of the unconscious into the conscious, and a new center of balance is obtained. There is a new location of the self, and Jung thought it provided a 'more solid foundation' for the psyche. Jung called this path to oneness *individuation*, although he did not see it as an easy journey. Much like Dorothy, we must face wicked witches on the path. Jung even characterized the process of individuation and therapy as one where the patient was forged between the hammer and the anvil.

Jung thought the process of individuation was also expressed as an arrangement or pattern in our dreams. If we made the conscious attempt to recognize the symbols in our dreams, we might become aware of our own grand pattern. However, this process, remember, might take years of studying our dreams. Images might appear, disappear, and reappear over a period of years. Many symbols may remain beyond us. However, if we actively and honestly search, Jung did believe that a slow, and perhaps even imperceptible, growth might occur, and this is the process of individuation. Yet, the product of this slow growth is a more stable personality, a more mature personality, and a new center of the self is established, one that is not so easily unnerved. A new, less anxious, less bored self emerges: a more reliant and more contented self, one that wants fewer material goods, one that is much happier with less.

Von Franz (1964) thought that Jung's self archetype might be symbolized in a dream by a 'priestess, sorceress, earth mother, or goddess of nature or love' or 'wise old man.' She suggested that a cosmic man or Great Man, like Buddha or Jesus, might also symbolize the self archetype. However, the self might also not take these shapes. She even noted that sacred stones may symbolize the self, because they have been revered for millennia in many cultures. She said that people even in modern society may pick up stones for no particular reason. People may be simply attracted by an unusual color or shape, and, for some, the stones hold a secret fascination. She gave the example of ancient Germans who thought that the spirits of the dead continued to live in their tombstones. Even the present custom of having tombstones may have arisen from this older belief. We also make monuments to great people out of stone. What do the black granite shapes of the Vietnam War memorial in Washington, D.C. symbolize? It is a good example of the sheer power and mystery of stone. The holiest of pilgrimage sites for a Muslim is Mecca where the house of Abraham and Sarah stands. In that house is a holy rock, one said to be sent by God for them to build their house.

Von Franz hypothesized that a stone may also symbolize the self archetype for the following reasons:

> For while the human being is as different as possible from a stone, yet man's innermost center is in a strange and special way akin to it (perhaps because the stone symbolizes mere existence at the farthest remove from the emotions, feelings, fantasies, and discursive thinking of ego-consciousness). In this sense the stone symbolizes what is perhaps the simplest and deepest experience – the experience of something eternal that man can have in those moments when he feels immortal and unalterable...or certain stones left by simple people on the tombs of local saints or heroes, show the original nature of the human urge to express an otherwise inexpressible experience by the stone-symbol. It is no wonder that many religious cults use a stone to signify God or to mark a place of worship.
> (Jung, 1968; p. 224)

When I taught in India for four months on a Fulbright Fellowship in 1987, I went hiking one weekend over a short but long stone hill. On the other side, I encountered a maze lined by pebbles and small stones in the form of a circle. In the center of the circle, stood a pile of stones about three or four feet high. Quite naturally, I picked a stone from well outside the circle, wound my way through the maze to the center pile, dropped off my rock, and proceeded back out of the maze. What it all symbolized, I have no idea nor did anyone I talked to when I returned to the sophisticated city of Bangalore. However, as Jung noted, that is the wonder and mystery of symbols. There is always some enigma associated with a symbol that may never be solved, and therein resides our eternal fascination for stones, circles, and mystery itself. Symbols, according to Jung, are representations of the unknowable.

The self archetype, like all other archetypes, possesses a good–bad duality. The dark side of the self is potentially the most dangerous, because the self archetype is the most important in the psyche. Von Franz describes the dark side of the self out of control or in a state of imbalance:

> It can cause people to 'spin' megalomanic or other delusional fantasies that catch them up and 'possess' them. A person in this state thinks with mounting excitement that he has grasped and solved the great cosmic riddles; he therefore loses all touch with human reality. A reliable symptom of this condition is the loss of one's sense of humor and of human contacts.
> (Jung, 1968; p. 234)

It is interesting to note cases of the dark side that have gotten out of control in contemporary society. A paranoid religious cult leader, James Jones, in 1978 led over 900 people to their deaths in a mass suicide-murder in South America. A Japanese cult leader, Shoko Asahara, also respected by his followers as being a divinely inspired savior, in 1995 had his followers murder 12 innocent train travelers with poison gas in Japan. David Koresh, an American religious cult leader, ended up dying along with over 70 of his followers and their children, in a 1993 raid of their 'religious' compound. It appears that all three 'religious' leaders had this megalomanic spin to their personalities. All three were directly associated with the deaths of innocent people, and all three had an undeniably magnetic ability to attract followers to their delusory fantasies. Although von Franz thought a reliable symptom of the dark self gaining control of a person's personality was a loss of human contact, it appears, sadly, that the opposite may be true in some cases.

The internal boredom that cult followers may feel initially, and perhaps the positive side of the self archetype in them, serves as the motivation for their search for an external leader to provide them with meaning in their lives. They fail to see that their quest, although noble and worthy, is an internal one. A guru can guide, but the problem for the guru and his or her followers is that the guru may become deified in the process. What fails to be recognized is that the roads the guru took for self-enlightenment can rarely be the same roads that anyone else can follow. This has disastrous consequences, as my previous three cult leader examples have shown. Von Franz wrote about how 'the evil spirit of imitation...makes one miss the target and...[one can] petrify psychologically.'

She further wrote:

> As I pointed out earlier, the process of individuation excludes any parrot-like imitation of others. Time and again in all countries people have tried to copy in 'outer' or ritualistic behavior the original religious experience of their great religious teachers – Christ or Buddha or some other master – and have therefore become 'petrified.' To follow in the steps of a great spiritual leader does not mean that one should copy and act out the pattern of the individuation process made by his life. It means that we should try with a sincerity and devotion equal to his to live our own lives.
> (Jung, 1968; p. 235–6)

Jung believed that modern people were too often bored, exhausted, and disenchanted, but the answer to their dilemma was the adventure within themselves. Getting in contact with their inner world through their dreams might be the answer to the ultimate meaning of life. Von Franz states:

> One gives one's mind, as before, to outer duties, but at the same time one remains alert for hints and signs, both in dreams and in external events, that the Self uses to symbolize its intentions – the direction in which the life-stream is moving.
> Old Chinese texts...often use the simile of the cat watching the mouse hole. One text says that one should allow no other thoughts to intrude, but one's attention should not be too sharp – nor should it be too dull. There is exactly the right level of perception.
> (Jung, 1968; p. 228)

Other archetypal themes

Jung was also fascinated by archetypal numbers. I previously mentioned the archetypal duality, symbolized by day and night, yin and yang, black and white, heaven and hell, devil or angel, good and bad, right and wrong, on and off, Adam and Eve, Ara and Irik, who are creator spirits of the Iban people of Borneo, Apsu and Tiamat, creator deities of ancient Babylonia, Rangi and Papa, creators for the Maori, and the Chinese creator Pan Gu who lived inside an egg for 18 000 years and then split into two parts creating the heavens and the earth, Mboom and Ngaan, two African creator deities, and easily thousands of other dichotomies. Woody Allen has said that there are only two types of people, those who categorize people and those who do not. At my college graduation in 1969, I remember only that the commencement speaker said people are tyrannized by categories. Yet, categorization itself masks a hidden archetype symbolized by numbers and the varying members in each class that each number represents.

Although Jung spoke of dualities and trinities, it appears that he was powerfully drawn to the concept of quaternity or fourness. He even called quaternity a 'strange idea' but noted how strong a role it played in religions and philosophies. He himself postulated four psychological functions and four stages of animus and anima development. He claimed that the self archetype was frequently symbolized by four-sidedness. He wrote of the four seasons, four directions (north, south, east, west), and the four evangelists in the Bible. He also noted that fourness was probably more ancient than the concept of trinity. In fact, he said that, in Christianity, the concept of trinity (Father, the creator, Son, the redeemer, and Holy Ghost, the enlightener) superseded quaternity. However, the Christian concept of trinity is the religious symbolization of even a much older religious trinity from the Hindu religion, which speaks of Brahma, the creator, Vishnu, the preserver, and Shiva, the destroyer. The Hindu trinity predates the Christian trinity by at least 1000 years (the concept of trinity is not mentioned in the Old Testament). In Aztec mythology, the primordial being, Ometecuhtli, gave birth to four creator gods.

It is even psychologically revealing to note how strong the archetype of quaternity thrust itself into Jung's own writing. For example, he thought that the Christian trinity was unconsciously being transformed into a quaternity by a fourth force. What did he (and he alone) postulate that this fourth force might be? A dark and evil anima!

Pentamerous is the adjective describing five parts. Interestingly, a pentagram, a five-pointed figure, has long been used as a symbol in the occult world. The negative associations with the number five are plentiful. In America, we have the Pentagon, a five-sided building in Washington, D.C. housing the armed services administration (although this is not inherently negative, it is ironic that the Pentagon does not house the Department of Education or the Department of Happiness). There were five rivers in the Greek mythological underworld. There were also five ages according to Greek mythology, and according to Aztec mythology there were five world epochs called the five suns. The number seven has perhaps been symbolized to an even greater extent than the numbers five or six. There was a famous memory paper in psychology that bore the title 'Seven (plus or minus two),' because it had been observed that seven entities (plus or minus two for most people) appeared to be the limit of what people could keep in short-term memory. Thus, local phone numbers are usually seven digits. There are seven days in a week. According to Greek mythology, seven warriors took part in the war between the two sons of Oedipus, and each led an army that attacked one of the city of Thebes' seven gates. Much later, the movie 'The Magnificent Seven' had seven gunfighters. Seven holy sages are frequently mentioned in Hindu mythology, and, according to Australian aboriginal myth, seven sisters wandered about Australia to escape a lecher. When they reached the sea, they leaped up into the sky to become the constellation the Pleiades. Interestingly, in Greek mythology, the seven daughters of Oceanid (a sea nymph) were being chased by Orion when Zeus turned them into stars to save them – and they formed the Pleiades.

Jung's explanation for flying saucers and aliens

In Chapter 5, I gave my explanation for belief in UFO abductions and paralysis. Jung (1969) believed that the empirical fact of the existence of aliens and flying saucers from outer space was not as important as the psychic fact that people strongly believed in them. This psychic fact reinforced Jung's view of archetypes and a universal collective unconscious. Thus, it may be said that Jung's attitude towards UFO reports might be similar to his view on dreams: they were credible because they might reveal the workings of and meanings in an individual's psyche, and these reports were consistent with his conception of a shared, universal psyche. Jung also thought that the consistent reports of the shape of flying saucers, round or mandala-like, might be psychic manifestations of the self archetype.

Summary

1 Jung's most accessible and last book, *Man and his Symbols*, presents his views and those of his most trusted colleagues about the nature of the psyche, personal unconscious, and universal collective unconscious.

2 Jung thought dreams could open the way to the founding of a general comparative psychology from which understanding of the development and structure of the human psyche could be gained.

3 Jung strongly rejected the notion of a glossary of universal meanings for dream images and themes.

4 Jung thought dreams transmitted unconscious impulses and reactions to consciousness.

5 Jung believed that dreams served a compensatory function; that is, dream messages were attempts to compensate for 'a particular defect in the dreamer's attitude to life.'

6 Jung felt that archetypes manifested themselves in dreams and that these themes and images gave humans a glimpse of their much older, ancient mind.

7 Jung believed that UFOs and flying saucers, regardless of whether they really existed, were psychic representations of the self archetype, and thus might be unconscious attempts to seek greater meanings in life.

CHAPTER 7

An introduction to Fritz Perls' dream interpretation techniques

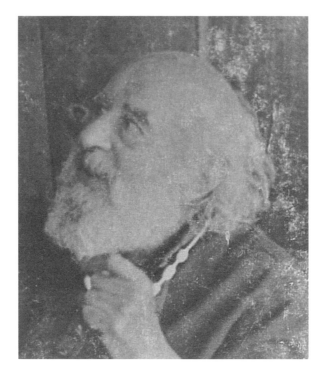

Figure 7.1: Fritz Perl

How can we fail to project ourselves into each and every dream thought? When we dream of our mothers, for example, is that dream image – as vivid and lifelike as it may be – really our mother? Is it really her words or script? Of course not. This tendency to project, however, is so strong that we often fail to realize we have done so. Freud postulated that *projection* was an unconscious ego defense, where we take unwanted or undesired self-traits and attribute them to others. Because the process takes place so quickly and automatically, we remain unaware that projection has even taken place.

I will give some examples. The first is a demonstration that has never failed in my general psychology class for over two decades. Look at the following two figures:

$$0 \qquad \Delta$$

Now, decide which one is happy and which one is out on parole for murder. Without any additional instructions and without any hesitation, 95% or more of every class decides that the circle is happy and the triangle is murderous. Then I stare at them in disbelief, while they typically giggle at their own folly. People, I say to them, these are drawings of chalk on a blackboard (or black ink on a whiteboard). They are not alive! They have no feelings, neither happy ones nor murderous ones. Then I point out that if they can project personality traits that easily upon the simplest of chalk drawings, imagine how more complicated our projections could be upon vivid dream images, and that includes both animate and inanimate images.

Another common example of projection occurs when we *anthropomorphize* (attaching human attributes to nonhuman things or animals). There was an eloquent story in a nonscientific magazine of a person who observed a funeral procession...among ants. The author courageously told the story of how the dead little worker ant was held aloft by its comrades in a solemn procession, carried sadly out of the main hole, and down the sides of the hill. Although scientists are not absolutely certain, it does not appear that ants are capable of anywhere near the same emotional sadness that humans feel. Furthermore, studies have shown that ants simply find the smell of a dead ant aversive (apparently the smell arises from decaying acids). In fact, if you take the decaying chemical and spray it on a live ant, that live ant will also be held aloft by its comrades and carried out of the anthill. People frequently anthropomorphize their pets, but it can be done as well with plants, cars, houses, or sports equipment. Again, if we can anthropomorphize animals, plants, or material possessions, imagine how easy it is for humans to attribute their own personality traits onto the vivid images in their dreams.

The modern discipline of behavior genetics has also shown that the largest factor contributing to the total sum of an individual's behavior comes from genetically based temperaments (e.g. Turkheimer, 2000). These temperaments are also mostly consistent across various situations and across one's lifespan (e.g. Heatherton and Weinberger, 1994). I believe that both factors may operate during dreaming. We probably project many of our deepest prejudices, biases, and offensive proclivities into our dream cast, script, and surroundings. Our dream themes will also be profoundly shaped by our ingrained, genetic predispositions to act and see ourselves act in very particular ways. Also, notice how these ingrained, genetic predispositions are consonant with Jung's notions of archetypes impelling behavior yet without a clear form.

It will be through dream interpretation that we will be able to become aware of these projections and underlying personality themes, and by becoming aware of them we will move toward solving issues and problems. Almost all of the types of psychotherapies operate on the principle that awareness is curative. Think about it. Have the reasons why psychotherapy works been explicated? No. We know how to do psychotherapy. We know that it takes extensive training and experience, but the *why* largely eludes us. Still, psychotherapies are generally successful. That has been empirically demonstrated. Some are better than others; some are better than nothing. Yet, most psychotherapies operate on the 'awareness is curative' principle. How ironic. Thus, as you learn about these dream principles and make patients aware of their unconscious issues, relax and have faith in the knowledge by which most therapies operate: awareness is curative.

Gestalt therapy

Fritz Perls (1893–1970) was one of the founders of *Gestalt Therapy*, and he was a lively and controversial figure of this popular psychotherapy of the 1960s. His early influences included German neurologist Kurt Goldstein and highly controversial neo-Freudian Wilhelm Reich. In Perls' book, *Gestalt Therapy Verbatim* (1969a), he outlined in only 71 pages its philosophical bases in a series of public lectures. Whereas Freud believed that dreams were the royal road to the unconscious, Perls thought that dreams served as 'the royal road to integration.' Dreaming, for Perls, was the most spontaneous thing that people do. He thought that language, specifically the things that we typically said, were mostly types of shit: *chickenshit* consisted of trite phrases like hello, how are you, etc.; *bullshit* occurred mostly in response to asking a person: *why?* Because Perls, like Freud, believed that psychic events were overdetermined, that is, they have many causes, there was no possible way that someone could come up with *the* answer to *why* they had done something. Finally, in his spontaneous and provocative humor, he added *elephantshit*, for which he gave Gestalt Therapy as an example, and he reserved the term for grand theories.

'So where was he coming from?' as we said in the 1960s. Well, Perls believed, much like Zen monks, in the sacredness of the here and now. He thought a neurosis, for example, did indeed produce the symptom of anxiety. However, for him, anxiety prevents growth. He said in a lecture at his California institute, Esalen:

> The stopping block seems to be anxiety. Always anxiety. Of course you are anxious if you have to learn a new way of behavior, and the psychiatrists usually are afraid of anxiety, they don't know what anxiety *is*.
>
> So the formula of anxiety is the gap between the *now* and *then*. If you are in the now, you can't be anxious, because the excitement flows immediately into ongoing spontaneous activity. If you are in the now, you are creative, you are inventive. If you have your senses ready, if you have your eyes and ears open, like every small child, you find a solution.
> (Perls, 1969a; p. 2–3)

Perls, much like Jung, also found that boredom was telling. For Perls, boredom resulted from blocking off genuine interests. Perls in his autobiography, *In and Out the Garbage Pail* (1969b), claimed that boredom even shaped his behavior as a therapist. It was boredom in therapeutic situations that motivated him to be obnoxious to people or be a caster of gloom. In other situations, he said it motivated him to flirt, be sexy, or to write his autobiography. In defense of Perls, he was nonetheless greatly loved despite his often gruff image and his putting of his patients in a 'hot seat' in front of hundreds of people. He actually believed in creative frustration, that is, placing people in situations that not only forced them into the *here and now* but also forced them to be real and not full of automatic trite phrases like, 'Hello, how are you?'

Topdog and underdog

Perls postulated another block to being able to live fully and freely was a war within the psyche between two parts which he called *topdog* and *underdog*. Perls imagined topdog as righteous and authoritarian (much akin to Freud's superego). Perls said topdog is 'sometimes right, but always righteous.' Topdog bullies our awareness with automatic prescriptions for living such as 'you should' and 'you should not.' Topdog also threatens our consciousness with demands and threats of catastrophe, such as 'you won't go to heaven if you don't do this,' etc. But Perls thought we have evolved a worthy adversary, underdog (akin to Freud's ego), who in some ways is even more dastardly clever. Underdog manipulates (or dominates) our awareness with being defensive, apologetic, and whiny. Underdog often defeats topdog by saying such things as 'I'm sorry,' and 'I tried but it's not my fault that I failed.' Also, underdog very cunningly places blame elsewhere and has us join organizations such as 'adult children of formerly abusive parents.' Perls firmly believed that even if you were hit with a potty chair in Cincinnati in 1957 by an alcoholic father, it is very well time to get over it. Perls believed that people should take responsibility for their actions right *now*. Perls felt that blaming others was unhealthy and blocked us from being psychologically free.

Perls thought that this self-torture game could even be carried to others. Perls noted that we usually automatically accept that topdog is always right and that we should be better humans, better children, better parents, etc. Yet, there is never any release from these demands for perfection from the topdog. Even if we have achieved some goal (e.g. perfect grades for a semester, getting a raise, etc.), topdog will immediately torture underdog with such lines as, 'Yes, but you'll never do that next semester,' or 'But you'll never get a raise that good again.' Furthermore, Perls thought that topdog always extends itself to others, and so we often berate others for failing to live up to our unreasonable expectations of them.

For Perls, these unrealistic expectations of ourselves and others are a damaging fantasy. Yet, he said, we take the fantasy for reality: it is an impasse. Perls believed that the impasse could be broken through a *satori* (insight). And this satori might come through some awareness of *how* we are stuck. Undoubtedly, Perls also believed that these satori could come through the most spontaneous expression of our existence – that is, dreams.

The Gestalt prayer

Although it has been taken out of context and even ridiculed, Perls reiterated his Gestalt prayer. It was not meant to be a moral code for evaluating all human behavior. Its primary purpose was to free people of the continual disappointment we feel in ourselves and others when we, and others, fail to live up to the unrealistic expectations of topdog. The Gestalt prayer is:

> I do my thing and you do your thing.
> I am not in this world to live up to your expectations
> And you are not in this world to live up to mine.
> You are you and I am I,
> And if by chance we find each other, it's beautiful.
> If not, it can't be helped.
> (Perls, 1969a; p. 4)

When freed of the self-torture game, we have a greater sense of awareness. Perls always emphasized *how* rather than *why*. He thought answers to *why* would simply perpetuate our anxiety created by the gap between *now* and *then*. It would also perpetuate our continued failure to take responsibility for our own actions. For example, an overweight adult might blame his or her alcoholic father for driving him or her to equate food with love. Perls fought strongly to abandon that blaming game and the search for a *why*. Perls thought it much better to live in the present. Of course, living in the *here* and *now* is a continuum. We cannot always ignore where we have been or where we are going. However, Perls was undoubtedly right: people can spend too much time worrying about the past and future and ruining a perfectly good present.

Here and now

The contemporary Vietnamese Buddhist monk, Thich Nhat Hanh (1991), stated this practice of the *here and now* eloquently and mundanely:

Washing dishes

To my mind, the idea that doing dishes is unpleasant can occur only when you aren't doing them. Once you are standing in front of the sink with your sleeves rolled up and your hands in the warm water, it is really quite pleasant. I enjoy taking my time with each dish, being fully aware of the dish, the water, and each movement of my hands. I know that if I hurry in order to eat dessert sooner, the time of washing dishes will be unpleasant and not worth living. That would be a pity, for each minute, each second of life is a miracle. The dishes themselves and the fact that I am here washing them are miracles! If I am incapable of washing dishes joyfully, if I want to finish them quickly so I can go and have dessert, I will be equally incapable of enjoying my dessert. With the fork in my hand, I will be thinking about what to do next, and the texture and the flavor of the dessert, together with the pleasure of eating it, will be lost. I will always be dragged into the future, never able to live in the present moment.

Each thought, each action in the sunlight of awareness becomes sacred. In this light, no boundary exists between the sacred and the profane. I must confess it takes me a bit longer to do the dishes, but I live fully in every moment, and I am happy. Washing the dishes is at the same time a means and an end – that is, not only do we do the dishes in order to have clean dishes, we also do the dishes just to do the dishes, to live fully in each moment while washing them.

(Hanh, 1991; p. 26–7)

Gestalt therapy ingeniously linked this spontaneity of dreams to the spontaneity of the *here* and *now* in therapy. Furthermore, Perls firmly believed, as most therapists, that awareness, per se, was curative. The use of dreams in Gestalt therapy helped the person become aware of their problems. However, as an existential therapy, the purpose of Perls' dream techniques was not simply to find a 'problem.' Perls believed that people were systems that sought balance. He felt that imbalances were perceived as a need for correction, and stated:

Now, practically, we have hundreds of unfinished situations in us. How come we are not completely confused and want to go out in all directions? And that's another law which I have discovered, that from the survival point of view, the most urgent situation becomes the controller, the director, and takes over. The most urgent situation emerges, and in any case of emergency, you realize that this has to take precedent over any other activity.

And I believe that this is the great thing to understand: *that awareness per se – by and of itself – can be curative*. Because with full awareness you become aware of this organismic self-regulation, you can let the organism take over without interfering, without interrupting; we can rely on the wisdom of the organism.

(Perls, 1969a; p. 15–16)

This notion of the inherent wisdom of the organism is consistent with the thinking of Carl Rogers (1902–1987), the humanist and founder of client-centered therapy. Rogers postulated a mental health motive, arising from the unconscious, that would impel people ultimately to correct themselves. That is why in therapy, a client-centered therapist had no need to advise, suggest, or cajole a client into what the therapist believed was the correct decision. The natural and inherent wisdom of the organism would self-regulate and self-heal.

How exactly does this healing process occur? The word 'gestalt' in Gestalt therapy means 'form.' Perls saw a law that he felt was constant in the universe, that is, the tendency for the world and every organism to maintain itself, and 'the only law which is constant is the forming of gestalts – wholes, completeness.' A gestalt was an 'organic function' to Perls. A gestalt was the 'ultimate experiential unit.' A patient in therapy or people in one of Perls' workshops would, through their dreams, project the 'holes' of their personalities onto the therapist. They would project their hierarchies of unfinished issues onto to the therapist. It would be the therapist's job to skillfully frustrate the patient to the point of confusion. The skillful part came where the therapist did not frustrate the patient to the point of depression nor let the patient get off too easily. Perls said:

> If you become aware each time that you are entering a state of confusion, this is the therapeutic thing. And again, nature takes over. If you understand this, and stay with confusion, *confusion will sort itself out by itself.* If you *try* to sort it out, *compute* how to do it, if you ask me for a *prescription* how to do it, you only add more confusion to your productions.
> (Perls, 1969a; p. 24)

Now, let us return to our original premise that everything in a dream is the dreamer and show how it is reflected in Gestalt therapy. Perls stated:

> Now if my contention is correct, which I believe of course it is, all the different parts of the dream are fragments of our personalities. Since our aim is to make every one of us a wholesome person, which means a unified person, without conflicts, what we have to do is put the different fragments of the dream together. We have to *re-own* these projected, fragmented parts of our personality, and *re-own* the hidden potential that appears in the dream.
> (Perls, 1969a; p.67)

I will explain the specific dream techniques with elaborate examples in later chapters. Presently, I feel it is necessary to explain the philosophy behind the techniques as a kind of prerequisite. The process of dream interpretation always reminds me of Jung's prescriptions for interpreting dreams:

> I have no theory about dreams, I do not know how dreams arise. And I am not at all sure that my way of handling dreams even deserves the name of a 'method.' I share all your prejudices against dream-interpretation as the quintessence of uncertainty and arbitrariness. On the other hand, I know that if

we meditate on a dream sufficiently long and thoroughly, if we carry it around with us and turn it over and over, something almost always comes of it. (Jung, 1970; p.74)

I especially like the imagery of turning a dream over and over. In what is probably my single favorite book *In Watermelon Sugar* by Richard Brautigan (1968; and not because it has a chapter entitled 'Fred'), the nameless hero meets Fred (his buddy) at dinner and relates the following:

Fred had something strange-looking sticking out of the pocket of his overalls. I was curious about it. It looked like something I had never seen before.
'What's that in your pocket, Fred?'
'I found it today coming through the woods up from the Watermelon Works. I don't know what it is myself. I've never seen anything like it before. What do you think it is?'
He took it out of his pocket and handed it to me. I didn't know how to hold it. I tried to hold it like you would hold a flower and a rock at the same time.
'How do you hold it?' I said.
'I don't know. I don't know anything about it.'
(Brautigan, 1968; pp. 6–7)

It makes me think the thing that Fred found might have been a metaphor for a dream. Contrast that dialogue with Jung's earlier writing:

One would do well to treat every dream as though it were a totally unknown object. Look at it from all sides, take it in your hand, carry it about with you, let your imagination play round with it, and talk about it with other people.
So difficult is it to understand a dream that for a long time I have made it a rule, when someone tells me a dream and asks for my opinion, to say first of all to myself: 'I have no idea what this dream means.' After that I can begin to examine the dream.
(Jung, 1970; p. 64)

Dreams form a hierarchy of unfinished business.

Fritz Perls thought dreams were the most spontaneous expression of human existence, and now we are at the crux of perhaps the most important dream principle in this book (in my opinion). First, to appreciate experientially the theory behind Gestalt Therapy and this important principle, please examine the following figure:

What is this figure? If you said a circle, you are wrong. It is a curved line. It was intentionally drawn to leave a very small space so that the circle was not completed. Perls argued that humans have a strong tendency to see things as whole objects or complete forms. The word Gestalt means *form*. Psychology students have long had to memorize the *Zeigarnik effect*, which states that unfinished tasks are remembered better than finished tasks. This effect appears to be particularly true for tasks which we take personally or when the tasks are ego-involving. For example, we worry about studying for an upcoming test. Whether we study for the test is another issue but we tend to think about studying for it a lot. The worry introduces itself into our consciousness continually. However, tests we have just taken and done well on we tend to forget, or they do not occupy nearly as much time as the tests we are about to take.

Now let us all recall the second part of Perls' argument:

> ...[A]ll the different parts of the dream are fragments of our personalities. Since our aim is to make every one of us a wholesome person, which means a unified person, without conflicts, what we have to do is put the different fragments of the dream together. We have to *re-own* these projected, fragmented parts of our personality, and *re-own* the hidden potential.
> (Perls, 1969a; p. 67)

Because of the phobic attitude, the avoidance of awareness, much material that is our own, that is part of ourselves, has been dissociated, alienated, disowned, thrown out. The rest of our potential is not available to us.

In summary, Perls suggested that our unfinished psychological issues form a hierarchy, or ranking. The unfinished psychological issues that are most important to us would move towards the top of the hierarchy and uncompleted psychological issues that were not as important would remain in the hierarchy, but at lower levels. The issues at the top of the hierarchy would be expected to make their way into our dreams repeatedly, perhaps by their recurrence in dreams. Thus, when listening to and helping a dreamer interpret their dreams, it would be important to first listen and form hypotheses as to what these higher-ranking psychological issues might be and then to help the dreamer become aware and re-own these fragmented parts of their personality. I will give numerous examples of how to accomplish the latter task in Chapter 11.

Summary

1 Dream images are probably replete with projections of our own personalities, unconscious and conscious issues and attitudes.
2 Fritz Perls, one of the founders of Gestalt Therapy, believed that dreaming was the most spontaneous of all human behaviors.
3 Perls thought anxiety was caused by a failure to stay in the 'here and now.'
4 Perls believed that all parts of a dream were projected fragments of our personalities.
5 Perls believed that our unfinished issues and problems formed a hierarchy which could be accessed through dream work.

CHAPTER 8

Troubled sleep and dreams

'How did you sleep last night?' must be one of the most often repeated morning greetings throughout the world. Indeed, sleep disorders and problems such as insomnia and disturbing dreams and nightmares are probably ubiquitous to all human beings and probably have been for millions of years. Furthermore, there is an undeniable link between sleeping well on a regular basis, and one's health and happiness (e.g. Dement and Vaughan, 1999). In fact, even how long we live is better predicted by adequate sleep on a regular basis than by diet and exercise.

The term 'insomnia' is a bit of a wastebasket category for many different types of sleep disturbances. It can describe difficulties with falling asleep, staying asleep, waking up during the night and failing to get back to sleep, waking up too early, or unrefreshing sleep. Of course, none of these problems are lethal but they certainly can be when, the following day, we are too sleepy and fatigued to stay awake in the course of our jobs or daily chores, like driving a car or truck, or operating heavy machinery, or when concentration and alertness are critical, such as for air traffic controllers, surgeons, or people who fix brakes on cars.

Whereas insomnia may seriously affect approximately 30–40% of a given population, disturbing dreams or nightmares will generally affect about 100% of a given population (lifetime prevalence rate). And disturbing dreams and nightmares can be another cause for insomnia. Some people fear going to sleep because of their anxiety about having bad dreams. In this chapter, I shall review the prominent types of sleep disturbance, including insomnia, disturbing dreams, and nightmares. I will also review various treatment approaches to these problems. In Chapter 10 I will also give examples of how bad dreams and nightmares can be examined and used in psychotherapy.

Insomnia

When a person or patient reports insomnia or being an insomniac, it could refer to many different kinds of problem, as was noted above. It therefore follows that insomnia cannot be defined by a given amount of sleep. The first problem in such a definition is that while the average amount a human sleeps is about 8 hours, some people feel fine and completely rested with only 5 hours sleep and some need 9 to 10 hours to feel good the next day. There is also a kind of stereotype that short-sleepers are more admirable and industrious while long-sleepers tend to be lazy. Empirical research has demonstrated that these biases are completely unfounded, as there are no demonstrated personality, physiological, or general health differences between natural short- and long-sleepers. Apparently, the basis for the variance in sleep length is strongly genetic as are the amounts of slow-wave (stages 3 and 4) and REM sleep (e.g. Toth and Verhulst, 2003). A genetic origin has even been found for a rare familial disease that make people suffer from perpetual jet lag (Ying Xu *et al.*, 2005). Thus, it may be summarized that some kinds of insomnia are genetically based, and it follows that some people who nearly always sleep well may also be genetically 'blessed.'

Besides the genetic bases for insomnia, there are obviously powerful environmental factors. One interesting one is taking a nap in the afternoon. Afternoon naps are more often filled with slow-wave sleep (Coolidge, 1974). Hours later, when these people attempt to go to sleep at the regular bedtime, their need for the deep, heavy slow-wave sleep has been relieved. They often interpret this as being unable to sleep, and they may further disrupt their regular sleep pattern by getting up, eating or drinking caffeinated beverages, which simply compounds their initial sleep problem. As just noted, caffeinated beverages may also prevent restful sleep. Alcoholic beverages in larger amounts tend to depress slow-wave sleep and REM sleep, and increase the number of sleep awakenings during the night, the latter of which interferes with the overall integrity of sleep. These forms of insomnia, where an external agent is the clear cause (e.g. caffeine, alcohol, etc.), are referred to as *secondary insomnia* because the problem is not directly related to another health problem or disease. The latter type of insomnia is called *primary insomnia*. Diseases like asthma, arthritis, and conditions where a person is in pain can cause primary insomnia. Mental states such as excessive anxiety, depression, and bipolar disorder are also frequently associated with primary insomnia.

Sleep experts also refer to acute and chronic insomnia. Acute insomnia generally passes quickly after a few days or weeks. People usually go back to their regular sleep patterns and suffer no long-term effects. Chronic insomnia is arbitrarily defined as affecting more than a couple of nights a week for at least a month. In the worst cases, people suffer from insomnia for years or even decades. Officially, the *Diagnostic and Statistical Manual of Mental Disorders* (*DSM-IV-TR*; American Psychiatric Association, 2000) defines primary insomnia as difficulty initiating or maintaining sleep, or nonrestorative sleep, for at least one month. According to *DMS-IV-TR*, the official diagnosis of insomnia requires that it significantly affect one's personal or occupational life.

So what is some general advice for dealing with acute and chronic insomnia? As noted earlier, the amount of sleep people need to feel rested varies. Over millions of years, humans have adapted their sleep–wake cycles to the 24-hour revolution of the earth. However, this adaptation is not perfect. Interestingly, in the absence of any time cues, humans' natural cycle seems to be slightly longer than 24 hours (Dement and Vaughn, 1999). One implication of this finding is that there is the possibility that all humans may sleep well for months at a time and then have difficulty sleeping for a while. This may occur because the underlying more natural 25-hour cycle becomes out of sync with the actual 24-hour revolution (day–night) cycle of the earth and sun. According to this theory, then, acute insomnia may wax and wane yearly on a rather regular basis. Thus, one treatment for acute insomnia may be just simple education. Nearly all people will suffer from acute insomnia at some time in their lives, and a majority may regularly but only periodically suffer from acute insomnia. Armed with this fact, we can simply accept the fact that insomnia is a very regular and natural part of our lives. If we do not sleep well tonight, perhaps we will sleep well tomorrow night or the next.

Some people, however, overreact to even brief periods of insomnia. If education and transcendence fail to help, there are over-the-counter and prescription medications. Of course, there are side-effects to this answer for insomnia, both physiological (e.g. feeling doped) and psychological (e.g. dependence) so it probably should be a last treatment of choice, although the temporary use of such medications can be fairly harmless for most people.

Other pieces of advice for dealing with insomnia are:

- Try to go to sleep at night and wake up in the morning at about the same time each night and day. As noted earlier, humans have natural sleep–wake cycles. The length of the cycles may vary somewhat from person to person; however, nearly everyone has a natural and consistent sleep–wake rhythm. Experiment to determine what your natural cycle might be. For example, I knew a psychologist/talk show host who fully recognized she was chronically crabby. After examining many other possibilities, it was suggested to her that perhaps she was not getting enough sleep. 'But I sleep a full eight hours!' she said, 'just like my husband.' After some experimentation, she was almost joyfully happy to discover that she needed nine hours of sleep, not eight like her husband.
- Naps are not harmful and are often helpful. However, remember that long naps (greater than one hour) in the afternoon often rob us of the need for stages 3 and 4 sleep when we finally go to bed at night. As a consequence, people who take a long nap in the afternoon often feel restless and suffer from insomnia when they attempt to go to sleep at night. In reality, they could just go to bed slightly later than usual, if they did take a long nap earlier. Naps can also be the *only* antidote to sleepiness when we are driving long distances (with the exception of amphetamines). Coffee or caffeinated drinks will only work temporarily or not at all. Recently, I have personally found that even a nap as short as 15 minutes restored me to nearly complete alertness while driving a long distance, and its effects completely warded off my sleepiness for the next six hours.
- Coffee, tea, and other caffeinated drinks should be avoided hours before bed-

time. Intense or heavy exercise hours before bedtime often interferes with restful sleep. Interestingly, heavy exercise early in the day will often increase the slow-wave stages of sleep (i.e. stages 3 and 4). This phenomenon may account for the folk myth that children who are observed to be highly active will sleep better at night. The myth actually has a basis in the relationship between exercise and slow-wave sleep, as long as the exercise is completed well before bedtime (as earlier noted). Smoking before bedtime (or anytime) is also harmful (for many other reasons) as nicotine serves as a stimulant and interferes with restful sleep.

- There is a physiological and evolutionary basis for sleeping in the dark. Thus, a dark place as opposed to a brightly lit place is much more advantageous for restful sleep. If you cannot control the amount of light in your sleeping place (e.g. on an airplane or as a passenger in a car), try a blindfold or sleeping mask. For some people, light-blocking makes a tremendous difference in the ability to go to sleep easily.

- There is no way to fully defeat jet lag. Diets that proclaim to defeat jet lag are completely fraudulent. Goggles and/or earphones that darken, lighten, or supply special sounds as one sleeps on a plane and purport to defeat jet lag are also completely bogus. It takes approximately three or four days, for most people, to adjust adequately to jet lag. It takes approximately two weeks for one's blood pressure and other physiological indices to return to normal when one flies to another country. The greatest jet lag occurs in trips to India (if one is from America), as they are almost exactly 12 hours the opposite, i.e. midnight in America is noon is India, and vice versa. There is no way to adapt to jet lag quickly and readily. Taking short naps while in a new country, supplemented by trying to adjust to the new country's typical sleeping and waking cycle as much as possible, is the only way to adjust to jet lag. I have found, for example, in my six trips from America to India, that I can start early before my trip, by sleeping later and staying up later, to aid in the transition. Also, when I arrive in India, I have found it much easier to succumb to naps (about 1–3 hours) than to try to fight to stay awake as long as possible, but I use both methods.

- If you cannot fall asleep easily, try to stay in bed and read, watch TV, listen to music, or engage in some activity that is not too exciting or overly stimulating. Try not to get out of bed, do housework, or rearrange your closet. Rest and relaxation is the next best thing to sleep, even if it is not sleep and will not substitute for sleep. Nonetheless, it is better than exercising or upsetting your normal sleep–wake cycle further.

Sleep apnea

The word *apnea* comes from Greek and means a lack of breathing. Sleep apnea occurs when people stop breathing or have trouble breathing while sleeping. In

DSM-IV-TR sleep apnea is classified under the rubric 'Breathing-Related Disorder'. By far the most common type of sleep apnea is *obstructive sleep apnea*. This type of apnea implies that something is blocking the trachea (windpipe). These obstructions tend to be more common in men (at a ratio of about 2:1 to 4:1) compared to women and seem to increase with age. The obstructions tend to be fatty tissue, relaxed throat muscles, tongue, tonsils, and other tissues. The more rare form of sleep apnea is *central sleep apnea*, and this form implies that the breathing problems are related to dysfunction in the central nervous system (CNS). Sleep apnea becomes a disorder when these periods of non-breathing, usually 10 to 30 seconds each, begin to disrupt sleep by waking a person up, or leave the person exhausted after a typical sleep period (e.g. 8 hours of sleep). As noted earlier, daytime sleepiness can have dire consequences when waking performance demands full alertness, e.g. driving a car.

Sleep apnea is very common in babies (nearly all will have some apneic episodes before the age of one), and it is not thought to be harmful. However, in some infants these episodes can extend for very long periods, like 30 seconds or more. Such episodes can leave a baby blue (from lack of oxygen) and limp. The latter form of sleep apnea is, of course, dangerous, and babies prone to this form may even have to be resuscitated or they may die. The exact relationship of this form of sleep apnea to *Sudden Infant Death Syndrome* (SIDS) is currently unknown. Some researchers, as I do, suspect that there is some relationship between the two. It may be more theoretically simplistic (fewer separate assumptions, which is a good thing) to assume that they are different forms of the same disorder. In its mildest and benign form, sleep apnea is common and nonpathological. In its mildest pathological form, sleep apnea episodes will last much longer than typical, and the babies may be left blue and limp. In its severest and most pathological form, SIDS, the infants will be found dead, and often there is no discernable heart problem or CNS disturbance. Recent empirical studies seem to link only maternal smoking to the pathological forms of sleep apnea in infants.

The following is some advice for those suffering from sleep apnea:

- One of the simplest and easiest ways to diminish sleep apnea is to try sleeping on your side instead of your back. People who sleep on their backs are far more prone to sleep apnea.
- Alcohol and sleep-aid medications appear to relax the throat muscles more than typical, thus resulting in more sleep apneic episodes. Try to reduce your dependence on alcohol or medications for sleeping.
- If you are over your ideal weight, lose some weight. Thinner people have fewer sleep apneic episodes, probably due to less fatty tissue obstructions in their throats.
- Have your sleep apnea evaluated by a certified or licensed sleep clinic that specializes in the disorder. In some circumstances, minor surgery is warranted and can be effective.

Narcolepsy

Narcolepsy involves sudden attacks of sleepiness while awake, and it comes from the Greek word *narco-* meaning numbness or stiffness and *-lepsy* meaning to seize. When narcoleptic people are monitored for their EEG waves, it is most often found that the sleep attacks consist of REM sleep. Compared to insomnia or sleep apnea, narcolepsy is relatively rare (about 7 cases in 10 000) although its symptoms can be dramatic. Sudden attacks of narcolepsy, which may occur 2 to 6 times a day, are often accompanied by muscle catalepsy, which is either a complete loss of muscle tone where the person may suddenly fall to the ground, or a partial loss of muscle tone where only the eyelids or head, jaw or arms may be affected. A little less than half of people with narcolepsy report an aura, which is a brief prodromal state that heralds the full narcoleptic episode. This aura may include dream-like hallucinations, which are also called *hypnagogic hallucinations*. As in normal REM episodes, narcoleptic people often report being paralyzed during their sudden REM onsets, which as previously noted in the book, is called muscle atony and normally accompanies nearly all REM sleep.

The cause of narcolepsy is strongly suspected to be genetic as it runs in families, and recent empirical work with dogs and humans suggests a complex inheritance pattern. It appears to occur equally for both genders. The waking narcoleptic attacks often interfere with the regular integrity and pattern of stages 3 and 4 and REM sleep. Thus, narcoleptic people very often feel sleepy during the day, in part, it is suspected, as a consequence of not getting REM sleep during their normal sleep period. Narcoleptic people often become anxious that they may suffer a bout while driving or during some other critical task. Thus, they may curtail many social activities and interactions with others for fear of having an attack.

There is no cure for narcolepsy but it does have some semi-successful symptomatic treatments. These treatment approaches are most often two-fold: prescription medications, usually CNS stimulants, and nap-therapy, which involves scheduling short naps three or more times a day in order to ward off sleepiness and impending narcoleptic attacks.

Other general advice for narcoleptic people is as follows:

- Education of narcoleptic people and their families about the nature and causes of narcolepsy often helps to reduce fears about narcolepsy and the stigma that may be attached to it. Learning about narcolepsy also helps others to avoid attaching pejorative labels such as lazy, unmotivated, or late-night-party person when the narcoleptic behaviors are observed.
- Although narcolepsy is not presently curable, it is a manageable disorder that allows people with it to be completely normal and productive human beings. The current treatment of choice includes selected short naps and CNS stimulants.

Nightmares

The word *nightmare* comes from Old English and refers to a female demon that visits at night. The lifetime prevalence of nightmares cross-culturally is virtually 100%, as no one seems immune to at least one troubling dream at some point in their lives. Nightmares officially become a disorder if they repeatedly awaken the sleeper and the subsequent anxiety associated with the nightmares causes significant social or occupational trouble during wakefulness. The most intense and troubling nightmares appear to occur in REM sleep, although fleeting images and thoughts that cause anxiety can occur in other stages as well (e.g. stage 2). Because a majority of REM sleep occurs in the last third of a sleep period, nightmares tend to be reported towards the end of an 8-hour sleep period, most often, then, in the early morning. The anxiety generated from intense nightmares can prevent sleepers from returning to sleep. If the nightmares repeat themselves, these sleepers can develop comorbid psychopathological states, such as anxiety, depression, irritability, and, of course, daytime sleepiness and loss of concentration and attention.

By about the age of 5 years old, approximately 50% of children will awaken their parents with the report of a nightmare. Most children appear to grow out of regular nightmares, and about 1% to 10% of adults have regular but occasional nightmares. Women report more nightmares than men.

Nightmares posed a problem for Freud and his postulate that *all* dreams were wish-fulfilling. In his 1920 book, *Beyond the Pleasure Principle*, Freud (1920/1990) reluctantly recognized that neuroses developing after traumatic experiences like war and early childhood sexual trauma were often accompanied by nightmares. Freud in 1920 wrote:

> This [dreams from traumatic neuroses] would be the place, then, at which to admit for the first time an exception to proposition that dreams are fulfillments of wishes... But it is impossible to classify as wish-fulfillments the dreams we have been discussing which occur in traumatic neuroses during psycho-analyses which bring to memory the psychical traumas of childhood.
> (Gay, 1989, p. 609)

For Freud, this phenomenon (nightmares) implied that there was something even more primitive and ancient than his proposed pleasure principle (i.e. seek pleasure, avoid pain) upon which the unconscious operated. Although he believed we evolved to the point where the current function of dreams was to fulfill wishes, he hypothesized that their original function might have been different. He proposed that the original function might have been a place where exceptionally strong traumas broke through the last line of defenses against anxiety of the ego. And he postulated that, in repeated nightmares, there was an instinctual compulsion to repeat, and this repetition was also beyond the pleasure principle though not entirely in conflict with it. To explain that seeming contradiction, Freud thought that the compulsion to repeat a nightmare might allow for the ego's eventual mastery of the traumatic memory.

For Jung, nightmares were largely compensatory, just like regular dreams. He gave the example of people who have too high opinions of themselves having the dreams of falling. Thus, nightmares might often point out deficiencies in one's personality and even herald dangers in one's future courses of action. A nightmare, according to Jung, created by our unconscious, might perceive and predict future dangerous events and pass this information on to the conscious. However, as noted in Chapter 6, he cautioned that while nightmares may warn us this way, nearly as often they do not. In his view, dreams and nightmares are just sometimes run by a benevolent agency. Yet, a 'mysterious' hand may also guide dreams and nightmares, and thus they may even serve as traps. Jung, like Freud, also recognized that if it were traumatic events that triggered 'reaction-dreams,' i.e. nightmares, then the nightmares could 'hardly be called compensatory.'

Nightmares and recurring trauma dreams are also thought to be among the common symptoms of Post-Traumatic Stress Disorder (PTSD). PTSD involves a person being exposed to a highly traumatizing event, typically outside the realm of regular experience, such as war, rape, and natural disasters, and the subsequent development of a confluence of psychological disturbances such as distressing and recurring recall of the event, a numbing of responsiveness to social and interpersonal interactions, and heightened arousal (e.g. hypervigilance). It has been noted (Barrett, 1996) that the dreams and nightmares of PTSD victims tend to be literal reenactments of the trauma, often with some unusual and horrible twist to the story that did not actually happen. It has also been suggested (Barrett, 1996) that as time passes and the symptoms of PTSD become less severe, that the reenactment dreams become more symbolized and begin to integrate regular waking events.

General advice for people with nightmares:

- As noted previously, children generally begin to experience some distressing nightmares by the age of 3 to 6 years old. Parents may ameliorate their children's anxiety and fears as a result of these nightmares by gently reassuring their children that the dreams were only dreams and that the events did not and will not really happen. Sometimes, it may help to tell the children that dreams are like cartoons, they happen but they are not real, and they cannot and will not hurt the child.
- There is very strong evidence that nightmares appear to be directly related to waking anxieties. In the case of children, parents may be able to thwart the occurrence of nightmares by allowing the children to communicate their fears or anxieties before the children go to sleep. Soliciting their fears and anxieties before children go to sleep may not be a good idea, but allowing a free exchange of the child's thoughts before sleep may be.

- The previous advice for children also holds for adults. Going to sleep with a major worry or concern may hasten troubling dreams. Talking to a loved one or trusted friend before sleep may be useful. For major concerns and troubles, psychotherapy may be a solution. In general, avoid dream interpreters but seek licensed clinical psychologists who may have a specialty in dream interpretation, like Freudian, Jungian, or Gestalt therapists. Also watch for licensed clinical psychologists who may be proponents of Clara Hill's model of dream interpretation. In my opinion, it appears to be empirically based, ethical, and scientifically sound (Hill, 1996).
- Education is nearly always a good policy. In other words, informing clients, patients, friends, and family who have nightmares that the dreams are transitory, have no ultimate meaning, and everyone has at least one or more in their lifetime, may go a long way in reassuring people and relieving their anxieties about occasional nightmares.

Night terrors

Psychologically, night terrors are typically much more terrifying than nightmares. People who have night terrors wake up screaming or crying. Night terrors can also be physiologically differentiated from nightmares because the former are thought to originate in slow-wave sleep as opposed to nightmares with an origin in REM sleep. Thus, night terrors usually occur in the first third of a sleep period whereas nightmares most often occur in the last third of a sleep period.

In terms of prevalence, night terrors are much less frequent than nightmares. About 3% of children will experience a night terror and less than 1% of adults will. However, due to the embarrassment, confusion, and amnesia that may accompany night terrors, the adult prevalence rate may be higher than estimated.

People with night terrors wake up screaming, crying, yelling, or incoherently babbling. These terrifying vocalizations are usually accompanied by motor movements such as flailing, punching, and attempts to get up and run away or flee, and people with night terrors can hurt themselves or others during their episodes. Clinicians have interpreted these actions as protective reactions to the terrors that the dreamer has just experienced. Interestingly, however, people with night terrors rarely report a single coherent dream story as they might after a nightmare. At best they report a fleeting or fragmented terrifying theme, but more often night terrors are not recalled at all. Many people with night terrors are amnesic for their whole night terror episode, particularly in the morning (or at the end of their sleep period).

The *DSM-IV-TR* official diagnostic label for night terrors is 'Sleep Terror Disorder'. As is standard in the *DSM*, in order to be a disorder people with night terrors must have their social or occupational functioning disrupted. This disruption often occurs because people with night terrors can become ashamed of their disorder and may curtail activities where sleeping over at someone else's house is required, such as sharing rooms during conventions, vacations, trips, and even more intimate social interactions such as sleeping with another person.

Advice for children and adults with night terrors:

- It has been conventional thinking (e.g. *DSM-IV-TR*) that night terrors in children are not a sign of comorbid psychopathology but that they are in adults. Indeed, most children who do experience night terrors do not seem to grow up with any more problems than children who do not. However, a recent anecdotal study of children with bipolar disorder found that the parents of the bipolar children reported their children had many more night terrors than would be expected. In adults, typical comorbid psychopathology includes PTSD, Major Depression, and Generalized Anxiety Disorder. Accompanying personality disorders might include dependent, schizoid, and/or borderline.
- It has been reported anecdotally that alcohol and sleep sedatives may increase the frequency of night terrors. Other semi controllable risk factors include sleep deprivation, fatigue, and intense stress. Genetics may also play a strong role in the development of night terrors, as a ten-fold increase of night terrors is said to occur among first degree relatives.
- Education, again, may play a crucial role in the reduction or prevention of night terrors. Reassurance of parents that the night terrors of children are highly unlikely to be an indication of any other type of psychopathology is a good policy. (Bipolar disorder in children is extremely rare; thus, while a significant proportion of children with bipolar disorder may have night terrors, very few children are ever diagnosed with a bipolar disorder.)
- In adults with night terrors, psychotherapy may be recommended, even for a single session, to reduce anxieties about night terrors and their repercussions but also to evaluate these adults for accompanying psychological disturbances.

Restless Legs Syndrome

The restless legs syndrome (RLS) has received increasing attention over the past decade. In RLS, people report that when they go to bed or are asleep, they have an overwhelming compulsion to move their legs, or their legs become disagreeably uncomfortable. People with RLS will often subjectively report that their legs have the feeling of something crawling on them or bugs or worms creeping under their skin, itching, burning, aching, or extreme leg restlessness. They may also report that their legs are full of pain and discomfort. This discomfort prevents sleep or disrupts sleep, and often leaves these people feeling sleep deprived, anxious, upset, fatigued, irritable, and disagreeable. RLS appears to be relatively common as it has been reported that anywhere from 2–15% of an adult population may experience RLS. It may be that the chronic prevalence rate may be closer to the former estimate and the single or limited form of RLS may be closer to the latter estimate. Current thinking has it that RLS primarily is a central nervous system disorder that can be exacerbated by psychological stress and other personality factors. There is also a strong suspicion that RLS has a strong heritable component as there is a high incidence of RLS among first degree relatives. RLS may also increase in prevalence in some people with iron deficiencies, neurological lesions of the CNS, pregnancy, end-stage renal failure, and with the use of some psychotropic drugs such as anti-depressants, anti-psychotics, and mood stabilizers. Caffeine has been reported to exacerbate the symptoms of RLS.

RLS may occur in children but it tends to be reported for the first time in young adults (<20 years old) far more often, although a majority of people with RLS report their first episode after 20 years old. Although not currently listed as an official diagnosis in the sleep disorder section of *DSM-IV-TR*, RLS should be considered a valid disorder if it disrupts the person's social life or occupational functioning.

Advice for the treatment of people with RLS:

*   If RLS reaches the level of a disorder, a medical referral to a primary care physician is probably best. There are medications that seem to improve the most severe cases of RLS, although they tend to be dopaminergics, that is, drugs that are primarily used to treat Parkinson's disease. However, there is no single drug that is universally prescribed on a regular basis. Some people with RLS seem to improve on opioids, but these drugs, like the dopaminergics, may have severe side-effects. Of course, the safest of drug treatments may be increasing iron intake to see if that alone helps.

Sleep walking

Walking during sleep is relatively common and most often benign. Somewhere between 15–40% of children have been reported to walk at least once in their sleep, and about 3% of all children are reported to sleep walk on a regular basis. Approximately 5–10% of adults have benign sleep walking episodes, and the prevalence of sleep walking disorders in adults is thought to be approximately 3% or less. Again, in order for sleep walking to qualify as a disorder, it must bring significant impairment to the sleep walker's waking life. Latter examples might include fears of sleep overs at a friend's house (in the case of children), sleeping with bed partners (as in adults), or other social or occupational disruptions.

Contrary to popular opinion, sleep walkers are not carrying out dreams. In sleep laboratories, sleep walkers arise in stages 3 and 4 sleep (delta waves), thus sleep walking usually occurs in the first third of a sleep period. My students usually appear amazed that people can rise up and walk during their sleep, as if it is a highly intelligent behavior. At some philosophical level it might be; however, sleep walkers' general level of responsivity to their environment is low, and complex human behaviors like elaborate language or conversations, reasoning, and higher level decision-making are completely absent. The most complex human behaviors observed during sleep walking are confined to walking, opening a refrigerator door, and upon very, very rare occasions driving a car. There is also the folk myth that waking a person very suddenly or shockingly from a sleep walking episode could be deadly for the sleep walker, and it is a myth. However, Miss Manners might tell us that it is rude to wake up anyone suddenly or surprisingly, and of course people with heart conditions might be highly vulnerable to sudden or shocking waking techniques.

Other dangers from sleep walking include choking while eating during a sleep walking episode, going outside, walking into the street at night, and tripping or falling downstairs. It is thought that stress may increase the likelihood of sleep walking and common internal stimuli like a full bladder. Genetic contributions to sleep walking are also strongly suspected.

Advice for dealing with people who sleep walk:

- Simple etiquette requires that sleep walkers be gently directed back to bed. They should not be rudely or shockingly awakened, although awakening them kindly and directing them back to bed is also good advice.
- Therapy may be indicated for chronic sleep walkers especially where stress is suspected as a precipitating factor.

Dream interpretation with people who have troubled sleep and dreams

Like Gestalt therapist Fritz Perls, I believe that regular dreams, nightmares, night terrors, and even the experience of insomnia can be successfully used in dream interpretation as a psychotherapeutic technique. Often just the mere act of sharing these experiences and feelings in therapy can be reassuring, comforting, and hope-giving. I do, however, believe that the interaction with a therapist, especially where the therapist uses some of the dream techniques from Freud, Jung, and Perls, can be highly beneficial. In Chapter 11 I give examples of interpreting recurring nightmares and an example of a woman who said she never remembers her dreams.

Summary

1 Insomnia is a term for a variety of sleep disturbances including difficulties with falling asleep, staying asleep, waking up during the night and failing to get back to sleep, waking up too early, or unrefreshing sleep.

2 Sleep apnea is the stoppage of breathing during sleep, and it can occur for a variety of reasons including increasing age, obesity, and genetics. Sleep apnea is common in infants although its relationship to SIDS is presently unclear.

3 Narcolepsy involves sudden attacks of sleepiness while awake. It is much less common than insomnia or sleep apnea, and it is managed well by drugs and environmental interventions.

4 Nightmares are highly prevalent and, for most people and children, are thought to be dependent on waking anxieties.

5 Night terrors are much more disturbing than nightmares and appear to originate during slow-wave sleep. They are far less prevalent than nightmares and are thought to occur regularly in less than 3% of children and 1% of adults.

6 Restless legs syndrome occurs in about 2–15% of adults and is experienced as an overwhelming compulsion to move one's legs or perceiving one's legs as disagreeably uncomfortable. There is thought to be a highly heritable component to the syndrome.

7 Sleep walking is relatively common and most often benign. Up to 40% of children have at least one episode and up to 10% of adults. Contrary to popular opinion that sleep walkers are acting out dreams, sleep walking is most often instigated during slow-wave sleep.

CHAPTER 9

The prophetic nature of dreams

Near the beginning of April, 1865, Abraham Lincoln had a dream that he heard crying in the White House. He dreamt that he got up and searched the rooms for the source of the crying. When he came to the East Room, he saw a coffin guarded by soldiers, and the corpse had its face covered. When he asked a guard who was dead, the soldier said, 'The President. He was killed by an assassin.' On April 15, 1865, Lincoln was assassinated by John Wilkes Booth in Ford's Theater in Washington, D.C. His body was later placed in a coffin in the East Room of the White House, and it was guarded by soldiers.

On June 28, 1914, Bishop Lanyi of Hungary, who had once been a teacher of the Archduke Ferdinand of Austria, woke up very early in the morning from a troubling dream. He saw his former pupil assassinated along with the Archduke's wife. He recorded the dream and said a mass for them. At 11.15 a.m. on the same day, in Sarajevo, Bosnia, the Archduke and his wife were assassinated by a Bosnian Serb, and their assassinations served as the impetus for World War I.

There is no question that stories such as these are legion throughout literature. Many turn out to be mere urban legends and become validated only through their re-telling. I cannot verify either of these two stories, although I have checked on urban legend websites. Nonetheless, regardless of whether they are true or not, it is a fact that extant literature contains many reports of prophetic dreams and that people commonly believe in them. In this chapter, I will review five possibilities for prophetic dreams, from the mundane (coincidence and probabilistic) to the divine and beyond (synchronicity).

The notion that dreams can be prophetic is probably prehistoric, and it certainly occurs as one of the most prominent and dominant of the very earliest interpretations of dreams. In the oldest written mythic epic, Gilgamesh takes his troubling dreams to his mother, Ninsun, and she interprets his dream as to mean that Gilgamesh was about to meet a new wild-man adversary Enkidu but that they would become friends and achieve greatness together. Not only is this the first record of a dream interpretation, but it provides evidence for the archetypal link between dreams and prophecy. Furthermore, from a Jungian perspective, we may represent Jung's classic concern with the individuation of the shadow archetype or his two-million-year-old man in all of us. The latter figure represents the idea that we are the products of at least two million years of evolution and that in all of us there is ancient wisdom. In a Freudian sense, Gilgamesh may be a metaphor for the unification of a maniacal ego with the wild drives of the id. Their resulting truce may represent the intrapsychic moral of the story, a healthy and productive psyche.

History of prophetic dreams

The ancient history of prophetic dreams also contains a strong link to war. Ashurbanipal, an Assyrian king who ruled from 668 to 627 B.C., left a great library of about 21 000 clay tablets. On the tablets is preserved the story of how the goddess, Ishtar, appeared to Ashurbanipal in a dream and predicted his victory in war the following day if he would honor her. Apparently, he did so, as he was successful the next day in battle. This dream was also particularly common among the Egyptian pharaohs. As mentioned in Chapter 3, Thutmose IV had a dream that the great sphinx at Giza had told him he would become ruler of Egypt. University of Chicago Egyptology Professor James Breasted noted that in the thirteenth century B.C., the great pharaoh Ramses' son, Merneptah, had a dream in which the creator god, Ptah, appeared as a gigantic statue, handed Merneptah a sword, and reassured him of victory against a large Libyan army. Merneptah defeated the Libyan army in a rout. In about 663 B.C., Tanutamon, an upper Egyptian ruler, invaded and conquered lower Egypt on the basis of a dream that told him he was about to become ruler of all of Egypt. Of course, these dream prophecies were usually aided by Egyptian armies of well over 20 000 men for a single battle.

Alexander the Great (356–323 B.C.) had a dream that he would conquer the city of Tyre. Apparently assured by the dream, he went on to conquer the city and then carried a famous dream interpreter with him for the rest of his battles. It is important to note that, for various reasons, we probably read about successful prophetic war dreams more than unsuccessful ones. Professor Breasted, for example, in his book *A History of Egypt*, listed the prophetically successful war dreams for three pharaohs (Thutmose IV, Merneptah, and Tanutamon), but there were no reports of dreams that did not come true (Breasted, 1912). However, we do have a few stories of unsuccessful prophetic dreams. Xerxes (519–465 B.C.), a Persian king, took over 300 000 men and over 800 boats in about 480 B.C. and attempted to conquer Greece based on his dreams that he would be successful in such an endeavor. Because Greece was not very important in the world at that time, Xerxes' dreams seem particularly curious. After 13 years of mixed success and failure, Xerxes finally withdrew to Persia.

Hannibal (247–183 B.C.), a Carthaginian, acted on a dream that told him he would conquer the Roman Empire. A young angel-like man appeared to Hannibal in his dream and showed him the Roman Empire in ruin. The young man told Hannibal to go and that his fate would be accomplished. With an army of 20 000 infantry, 6000 cavalry, and 38 remaining elephants (after crossing the Alps), he invaded Italy with some initial successes in 218 B.C. However, through tough winters, poor provisions, insufficient help from his homeland Carthage, and local loyalties to Rome, Hannibal finally abandoned his Roman campaign. Hounded by Roman armies, Hannibal committed suicide by poisoning himself in about 183 B.C.

The use of dreams to prophesy has been a cross-cultural phenomenon since recorded history. It is not difficult to gather thousands of examples, not only from the world's literature but also we could do as well gathering this type of dream from friends and family members.

I think it is often a mistake to overlook the obvious. Thus I think it silly to question whether these prophetic dreams occur. They certainly do, and they are common, ancient, and universal. However, an important question we might ask is *why* do they occur.

I have previously mentioned incubation dreams of the early Mesopotamians and later the Egyptians. Van de Castle, in his book *Our Dreaming Mind*, notes the Greeks had refined dream incubation into 'a highly developed art' (Van de Castle, 1994). He wrote:

> The person seeking a healing dream went through rather elaborate preparatory procedures, which varied from temple to temple. Generally the person had to refrain from sexual intercourse, follow a special diet, and engage in frequent cold water bathing. Animal sacrifices were made and the dreamer would sleep upon the skin of the animal sacrificed, which was often a ram. Evening prayers or hymns were held during the 'hour of the sacred lamps,' at which time the supplicants would beseech Aesculapius (an earlier Greek healer) to provide them with their desired dream. Within the temples were statues of the god and testimonial plaques from previous visitors regarding their healings... After the torches were extinguished, priests would move about among the expectant devotees with words of encouragement.
> (Van de Castle, 1994; p. 62)

Van de Castle noted that all of these procedures obviously created conditions that would contribute to successful dreams. Apparently, the priests began to play increasingly important roles as dream interpreters and offered suggestions for cures to medical illnesses in particular. Hippocrates (469–399 B.C.) may have been the first of the Greeks to expound clearly on the types and functions of dreams. In a short essay, *On Dreams*, Hippocrates expressed a belief in prophetic dreams and in what might be considered a subtype of the prophetic dream, the *prodromal dream* (derived from the Greek word *prodromos*, which means 'running before'). Prodromal dreams present early symptoms of future diseases.

Hippocrates speculated on the possibility that bodily problems could be diagnosed through dreams and offered probably the earliest observation that 'all dreams are wish-fulfilling dreams' when he wrote: 'All the objects we believe to see indicate a wish of the soul.' This hypothesis upstages Freud by about 1900 years.

In a similar vein, Plato (427–324 B.C.) preempts Freud's id and Jung's shadow when he wrote: 'In all of us, even in good men, there is a lawless wild beast nature which peers out in sleep.' (Van de Castle, 1994; p.64). Aristotle (384–322 B.C.) was a highly astute observer when it came to sleep, dreams, and prodromal dreams. He wrote three short books, *On Sleep and Sleeplessness, On Dreams,* and *On Prophesying by Dreams.* First, he argued against his teacher Plato's belief (and against Hippocrates' belief) that astrology had anything to do with dreams. Second, he did not believe in dreams inspired by gods. His argument against the latter is an interesting one. He wrote that divinely inspired dreams were not likely, because these dreams appeared to common people. It certainly would have been interesting to have been able to ask Aristotle why the gods would have reserved their messages for important people only. Third, Aristotle presented the still reasonable theory that we sleep to conserve energy. His argument is a brilliant one, nevertheless, for it also presages adaptation and evolutionary theories. He wrote:

> ...as we assert that Nature operates for the sake of an end, and that this end is a *good*; and that to every creature which is endowed by nature with the power to move, but cannot with pleasure to itself move always and continuously, rest is necessary and beneficial; and since, taught by experience, men apply to sleep this metaphorical term, calling it a 'rest': we conclude that its end is the conservation of animals.
> (Aristotle, 1952b; p. 706)

Fourth, he was highly observant about the presence of sleep in living nature:

> Accordingly, almost all other animals are clearly observed to partake in sleep, whether they are aquatic, aerial, or terrestrial, since fishes of all kinds, and mollusks, as well as all others which have eyes, have been seen sleeping. 'Hard-eyed' creatures and insects manifestly assume the posture of sleep; but the sleep of all such creatures is of such brief duration, so that often it might well baffle one's observation to decide whether they sleep or not.
> (Aristotle, 1952b; p. 706)

Fifth, he noticed that 'infants, for example, sleep a great deal,' although for his reasoning he adopted a similar posture to Hippocrates about blood flow, temperature, and evaporative spirits moving up and down the body. This same incorrect reasoning led him to the correct conclusion that wine was not good for children or their wet nurses. Sixth, partially consistent with modern thought, he stated that: 'A person awakes from sleep when digestion is complete,' and, indeed, as stated in Chapter 2, the parasympathetic nervous system predominates during stage 4 sleep, and vegetative functions like digestion become much more active.

Another one of Aristotle's interesting passages was:

Nor is every presentation which occurs in sleep necessarily a dream. For in the first place, some persons [when asleep] actually, in a certain way, perceive sounds, light, savour, and contact; feebly, however, and, as it were, remotely. (Aristotle, 1952b; p.706)

There is also an earlier passage in this same work where Aristotle presented a similar thought; that is, not all thoughts or images that occur during sleep should be called dreams. This distinction was not made clear until late in the twentieth century, and indeed many still blur the distinction between thinking and imagery, between non-REM and REM sleep. Also, from this passage, it seems clear that Aristotle was also presaging the modern notion that our sleeping brain is not resting but, in some aspects, remains highly active. He did, however, go on to describe the incorporation of external stimuli into sleeping cognition as distinctly different from dreaming, and this may not be the case, although the issue is debatable.

While all of these observations are acute and commendable, I began this review on thoughts about prophetic, divine, and prodromal dreams. It is at this point that Aristotle becomes most relevant. He wrote:

As to divination which takes place in sleep, and is said to be based on dreams, we cannot lightly either dismiss it with contempt or give it implicit confidence. The fact that all persons, or many, suppose dreams to possess a special significance, tends to inspire us with belief in it [such divination], as founded on the testimony of experience... Yet the fact of our seeing no probable cause to account for such divination tends to inspire us with distrust. For in addition to further unreasonableness, it is absurd to combine the idea that the sender of such dreams should be God with the fact that those to whom he sends them are not the best and wisest, but merely commonplace persons... Well then, the dreams in question must be regarded either as *causes*, or as *tokens*, of the events, or else as *coincidences*; either as all, or some, of these, or as one only. I use the word 'cause' in the sense in which the moon is [the cause] of an eclipse of the sun, or in which fatigue is [a cause] of fever; 'token' [in the sense in which] the entrance of a star [into the shadow] is a token of the eclipse, or [in which] roughness of the tongue [is a token] of fever; while by 'coincidence' I mean, for example, the occurrence of an eclipse of the sun while someone is taking a walk; for the walking is neither a token nor a cause of the eclipse, nor the eclipse [a cause or token] of the walking... Are we then to say that some dreams are causes, other tokens, e.g. of events taking place in the bodily organism? At all events, even scientific physicians tell us that one should pay diligent attention to dreams, and to hold this view is reasonable also for those who are not practitioners, but speculative philosophers...for example, dreamers fancy that they are affected by thunder and lightning, when in fact there are only faint ringing in their ears...or that they are walking through fire, and feeling intense heat, when there is only a slight warmth affecting certain parts of the body. When they are awakened, these things appear to them in their true character. But since the beginnings of all events are small, so, is clear, are those also of the diseases or other affections about to occur in our bodies. In conclusion, it is manifest that these beginnings must be more evident in sleeping than in waking moments.

Nay, indeed, it is not probable that some of the presentations which come before the mind in sleep may even be causes of the actions cognate to each of them...the cause whereof is that the dream-movement has had a way paved for it from the original movements set up in the daytime; exactly so, but conversely, it must happen that the movements set up first in sleep should also prove to be starting-points of actions to be performed in the daytime, since the recurrence by day of the thought of these actions also has had its way paved for it in the images before at night. Thus then it is quite conceivable that some dreams may be tokens and causes [of future events].

Most [so-called prophetic] dreams are, however, to be classed as mere coincidences, especially all such as are extravagant,..

On the whole, forasmuch as certain of the lower animals also dream, it may be concluded that dreams are not sent by God, nor are they designed for this purpose [to reveal the future]. They have a divine aspect, however, for Nature [their cause] is divinely planned, thought not itself divine. A special proof [of their not being sent by God] is this: the power of foreseeing the future and of having vivid dreams is found in persons of inferior type, which implies that God does not send their dreams...they just chance to have visions resembling objective facts, their luck in these matters being merely like that of persons who play at even and odd [a game of chance].
(Aristotle, 1952c; p. 707–9)

Possibilities for the causation of prophetic dreams

Mere coincidence

Among these many ideas, I would like to summarize five possibilities for prophetic dreams starting with Aristotle's work. First, we have the possibility that prophetic dreams that come true are *mere coincidences*. This seems obvious and intuitively reasonable. We may dream of hundreds of ideas, people, thoughts, and images even within a month's worth of sleep. After a few years, one of these ideas comes true. We are filled with wonder despite the 999 dream ideas that did not come true.

Prodromal dreams

Second, we have the sophisticated Aristotle's notion that waking thoughts continue into sleep and sleeping thoughts may carry over into wakefulness. As Jung argued over 1900 years later:

> Thus, dreams may sometimes announce certain situations long before they actually happen. This is not necessarily a miracle or a form of precognition. Many crises in our lives have a long unconscious history. We move toward them step by step, unaware of the dangers that are accumulating. But what we consciously fail to see is frequently perceived by our unconscious, which can pass the information on through dreams.
> (Jung, 1968; p. 36)

I would argue that *prodromal dreams* may be a specific subtype of this category of dreams that interact with our waking thoughts and confirm Aristotle's notion that 'the beginnings of all events are small,' especially in diseases. For example, recently, a mother of five children heard I was writing this book, and told me: 'I had an interesting dream. The night before I miscarried a child, I dreamt I had had my baby, but I lifted him up and handed him to an angel. Later that morning, I had my miscarriage.'

In my 1983 study, *Dreams of The Dying*, my student, Cynthia Fish (whose father was an oncologist), had gathered dreams from 14 cancer patients, all of whom subsequently died of cancer. We had dreams for some of the patients from about six years up till about one month before they died. We found, not surprisingly, that death themes were quite frequent for about half of the group, and death themes occurred significantly more often than in a control group of physically healthy elderly people (who phenomenologically also face death). We also found that the cancer patients projected their death themes onto other dream characters more than about 85% of time.

In one tragic example, I had a student tell me that he had the recurring dream that his teeth were falling out. As we completed a literature search, we found that the dream was reported as far back as perhaps about 1750 B.C. Most fixed or glossarial interpretations portended death. We then found 14 college students who had his same recurring teeth-loss dream and tested them psychologically compared to a control group of 'flight' recurring dreamers. We found that the teeth dreamers were significantly more depressed and felt less in control of their lives than the control group. Five years later, this same student died in a car rollover in the mountains. Before anyone who has had this teeth-loss dream begins to panic, let me firmly restate my premise (and Jung's) of Chapter 6: *there is no standard glossary of meaning for dreams.* Also, I could not replicate these findings in a much larger study of college students with the teeth-loss dream (Coolidge and Salk, in press). However, this particular student was an outgoing, brilliant but sometimes erratic, risk-taker. His female peers affectionately called him a 'bad boy.' It was clearly part of his charm. Remember, Jung said that dreams can warn us of situations long before they happen, and we may be consciously 'unaware of the dangers that are accumulating.' So, he always drove without wearing his seat belt. It was dark. He was driving in the mountains. Like Jim Morrison of the Doors, one can tempt death only for so long.

Probability estimators

A third cause for prophetic dreams is that there is overwhelming evidence that dreams cannot only solve problems, or inspire us to creativity, but also our dreams may serve as *probability estimators*. By this, I mean that we frequently explore themes in dreams that we would never or rarely entertain in real life, and some of these are taboo thoughts. For example, I had a vivacious, red-haired aunt (my mother's youngest sister). One night, I dreamt she and I went riding on my motorcycle, with her arms and body clutched tightly to mine, and I also remember vividly that she was wearing a lime-green halter-top, as we drove about with the wind streaming through our hair. My brother was nearly physically sickened when I told him the dream (perhaps it was too much for a carpenter living in the rural hills of Georgia). I will admit that I had entertained a very fleeting sexual fantasy or two about her in my waking life. My unconscious REM state, in good Aristotelian fashion, picked up on these semi-conscious and unconscious issues and played out a more full 'what if?' in my dreams.

I think if we return to my first two opening examples in this chapter, we may be able to explain some prophetic dreams on the basis that they are not just instances of coincidence but that they are high probability events. It would not be unlikely that a president or leader of any country might have conscious and unconscious worries about being assassinated. It would not be unusual for these worries to be converted into dreams. We might postulate the same mechanism as previously discussed – REM as a probability estimator. In a ruler's conscious waking life, they may not wish to entertain the conscious fantasy of being assassinated, but dream sleep respects no such boundaries. The things we repress, fear, loathe, or are forbidden may all be dealt with during dream sleep. One example occurs in my office at the university on a semi-frequent basis. A male student usually walks in, looks furtively about, and sits down reluctantly. 'I have this dream,' he sputters. His ambivalence in telling me is all too evident. 'Let me guess,' I think to myself, 'you dreamt you touched another male.' Invariably he says, 'I dreamt I touched another male.' In my large general psychology class, I ask: 'Males. Does it feel good to touch another male?' A great silence always falls upon the classroom. Of course, it does. You can hug your brother like a bear.

He will not break. He hugs you back with gusto. It feels good, but we males will not walk around discussing the pleasures of hugging or touching other males, even though we do hug and touch. Thus, in dream sleep, without self-criticism, self-loathing, or self-judgment, we will explore the theme, 'I wonder what it would be like to touch another male.' For gay males, a similar disturbing theme might occur, 'What would it be like to touch a female?'

Divine inspiration

The fourth possibility for prophetic dreams is that they may be *divinely inspired*. This topic was covered in Chapter 3. Aristotle, just like Jung, does not entirely rule out the possibility that some dreams may be divinely inspired. As Aristotle logically argued, this type of dream's universality makes it compelling. As Jung argued, we are simply not listening. We are too caught up in the products and thinking of rational waking consciousness. It also reminds me, not only of Jung's rabbi who said no one today can bow low enough, but also of the humanist Abraham Maslow (1907–1970) who coined the term 'the Jonah complex.' Maslow would ask his students who among them would be the next president, brain surgeon, or Nobel Prize winner. When no one typically raised their hand, he said, 'If not you, who?' His point was that they were acting like Jonah when God asked him to do something. Jonah felt too humbled to be able to do anything for God. Whereupon, Jonah was swallowed by a whale for three days, then spit up on the beach. The next time God asked Jonah for something, Jonah had learned his lesson. Do not be too humble. Aspire for greatness. Listen to God speaking. If not you, who?

For argument's sake, let us take the other position that no dreams are divinely inspired, either because there is no God, or because God is dead, or because God does not communicate through dreams. This hypothesis certainly should change the theoretical foundations of many religions, although I suspect that because religion and God are largely acts of faith, it probably would not change the actual practice of any religion. It would logically mean that many current religions were founded on hallucinations, delusions, or simply on the basis of one person's random pons-lateral geniculate nucleus occipital lobe electrochemical spikes. For some reason, the latter is more frightening to me than the former (hallucinations or delusions). Interestingly, in mental hospitals, patients' hallucinations and delusions are often of an excessively religious nature.

Synchronicity

The fifth and last of my explanations for prophetic dreams comes from Jung, although I suspect its theoretical roots were established by Aristotle. This Jungian hypothesis is known as *synchronicity*. In its simplest form, Jung proposed, 'Even inanimate objects cooperate with the unconscious in the arrangement of symbolic patterns.' For an example, he gave the frequent anecdotal reports of clocks stopping at the exact moment that their owners have died or mirrors breaking upon a death in the household. Certainly, our only other scientific option is to explain these occurrences through coincidence, because even current science has one basic rule by which we know and understand phenomena: the law of cause and effect. Jung has proposed, however, a second law: synchronicity, which stated that external events could be connected to internal events through nonvisible means. Jung also used the term *meaningful coincidence* to describe this relationship. Examples from our daily lives are plentiful, although Jung thought they were more likely to occur when we were in the throes of an emotional crisis or during a crucial phase of our self-growth or individuation. Jung also thought that the synchronistic events were triggered by an archetype in the collective unconscious.

A common example of synchronicity might be when we go to telephone a distant relative or friend, the phone rings, and it is them, or when we go to call them or they us, and the other says, 'I was just thinking about you. I was just about to call you.' Jung himself had a dramatic example in his private practice. He was seeing a depressed man in therapy, and while Jung left town for the weekend, he suddenly awoke with a strange and foreboding feeling that something was wrong with his patient. When he returned to his practice, he found out that the man had killed himself virtually within minutes of when Jung was suddenly awakened from sleep. On the surface, it may appear that this is another instance of coincidence, but Jung argued that these were meaningful coincidences connected to each other (i.e. Jung's unconscious thought that the patient was in serious trouble, and the patient's suicide) but acausally.

Recently in one of my dream seminars, a woman about 30 years old asked me about the possibility that dreams that do come true are simply high probability events. She told me that she had a recurring dream of fuzzy, hairy animals. She said that invariably when she had the dream some disappointment followed. She said some relative confirmed that this was true about furry animal dreams in their family. However, she said she remained skeptical, because she knew that no one has to wait long for some disappointment in his or her life. Then, she asked me how I would explain the following dream, which she described as her most intense of all furry animal dreams.

> Two furry little rats came up and were biting my toes. I was trying to pull away but I could not. I woke up scared. It was 4 a.m. At 6 a.m., the phone rang. My fiancé had been killed that morning in a car wreck.

I told her I would not be inclined to explain her dream through probability estimation but through the concept of synchronicity, and I proceeded to explain this Jungian concept of meaningful coincidences.

It is also fascinating to think either that Aristotle came perilously close to describing the same phenomenon when he described tokens in dreams or that he actually did describe the principle of synchronicity. Aristotle's logical explanation of how tokens have an association to the causal event, because waking actions pave the way for dream images, and vice versa, is at least as coherent an argument as Jung's.

Summary

1   It is possible that prophetic dreams are merely coincidental. Out of thousands of our dreams, one comes true: big deal.

2   Prophetic dreams may be explained by Aristotle's notion that waking thoughts continue into sleep, and sleeping thoughts may carry over into wakefulness. Prodromal dreams may be a specific subtype of this category of dreams consistent with Aristotle's proposal that 'the beginnings of all events are small,' especially in diseases.

3   A third cause of prophetic dreams might be that our dreams may serve as probability estimators, that is, we dream of many possible outcomes for our future courses of action, and sometimes we follow one of theses courses.

4   A fourth possibility for prophetic dreams is that they may be divinely inspired. Theists would have a very tough time rejecting the notion that God could speak through dreams because the typical notion of a god is that He is all-powerful, and who could purport to know the mind or will of God? Atheists would simply dismiss the notion of divinely inspired dreams.

5   A fifth possibility for prophetic dreams comes from both Jung and Aristotle. The Jungian hypothesis is known as synchronicity or meaningful coincidence. According to Jung, dreams may sometimes portend the future because events can be related beyond simple cause and effect. Aristotle also proposed that dreams may indeed contain tokens that may portend future events.

CHAPTER 10

The recurring nature of dreams

A majority of people report having the same dream or dream theme over and over. Some say their repeating dream started in childhood while others report a later onset. Van de Castle (1994) has noted that earlier onset recurrent dreams are more likely to be disturbing while later onset recurrent dreams are more likely to be pleasant. There is also a category of dreams that Freud called *typical dreams* that may be highly recurrent although people may not report them as such. Typical dreams include themes of flying, falling, being chased, not being prepared for an examination, appearing nude or not dressed appropriately, or losing one's teeth (this latter dream may be one of the oldest written, appearing in an Egyptian papyrus in about 2000 B.C.). It appears that the research definition of recurrent dreams is vague and thus some people report they do not have recurrent dreams but say, yes, they do have frequent dreams of flying or falling.

Freud

Freud defined recurrent dreams as a dream which is 'first dreamt in childhood and then constantly reappears from time to time during adult sleep.' Curiously, he added, 'though I have never myself experienced one.' Apparently Freud's interest in recurrent dreams was only that they served as evidence that dreams contain impressions from childhood that do not appear to be accessible to waking memory. Also curiously, Freud reported at least two dreams about his friend Otto in *The Interpretation of Dreams* and provided his readers with elaborate interpretations of Otto, yet Freud did not define Otto as a recurrent dream theme.

I am making these observations about recurrent dreams for two reasons. One, it is clear that the percentages of people reporting recurrent dreams will vary widely depending upon the dream researcher's definition and the way in which this question is worded to the subjects. Second, I am fascinated with Freud's dreams of Otto because of my own recurrent dream for the past three decades. I have dreamt of a buddy from Catholic school whom I met in the fifth grade, although the dream has declined in frequency from about once a month to once a year. The recurrent theme of the dream is that I see him (we both continue to age normally) but he will not talk to me. In real life we were close friends from fifth grade through about ninth or tenth grade when I developed other friends and interests. By my senior year of high school we rarely spoke, although I had not made any conscious decision to drop him as a friend. We both went to different colleges. By graduate school, however, he was appearing in my dreams so frequently that I decided to find out where he was, look him up, talk to him, and get him out of my dreams. I soon learned that he was transferring to my university. Within the year, I called him up and arranged for a meeting with him and another one of our mutual friends from high school. As I left my apartment, I told my wife, 'This is it. He's out of my dreams after tonight.' As soon as I met him, I knew he was not the fellow in my dreams. It was his face, it was his name, but the fellow I had internalized a long time ago was not the same fellow who sat before me. Nevertheless, I tried renewing our friendship but we had grown into different people, and I never saw him again except in my dreams.

According to Van de Castle, there is a consensus among clinicians that if one solves the underlying psychological enigma, then the recurrent dream will end. For about the past 15 years, in my dream interpretation workshops, I have presented my dream first, both to loosen the audience up by sharing with them and to get their help in solving the meaning of my dream. With only some decrease in frequency, however, my dream of my old buddy reappears now at least yearly. My suspicion is that, like Freud and Jung, dream images may carry more than one meaning (overdetermination), and that this fellow in my dreams (me) represents more than one issue, like my own strong feelings about friendships, aging, and loss. Interestingly, as I write this, I am suddenly reminded about a conversation with my recurrent dream buddy that we had in the eighth grade lunchroom. I was turning 14 that year (he was about 10 months younger), and I remember telling him alarmingly that we were aging and dying right before everyone's eyes yet no one seemed to care. 'Fred,' he said, in a blasé manner, 'there's nothing you can do about it.'

Sagan

Carl Sagan, an astronomer, thought that recurrent, typical and frightening dreams replay our ancient evolutionary history. For example, he noted that there appears to be only three genetically controlled inherited fears in most young primates: fear of falling, fear of snakes, and fear of the dark. He linked these fears to our early evolutionary history when our earliest ancestors were tree-dwellers (the youngest of human infants can still be lifted from the ground by the strength of their grip, which may be an ancient reflex for holding on to our ancient ancestral mother's hairy body). He also links them to an ancient evolutionary competition between mammals and reptiles (like snakes). Interestingly, a reptile, the snake, leads to the downfall of Adam and Eve in the Bible. Finally, Sagan links these dreams to fears of night predators, which cannot be seen well in the dark. This latter example strengthens Webb's argument that we evolved sleep to protect us from wandering around and falling prey to dangers in the night.

It is also interesting to speculate about the three other typical dreams we have not yet explained, the examination dream, appearing nude, and the loss of teeth. The examination dream, which Freud described elaborately in *The Interpretation of Dreams*, usually involves the dreamer not being prepared for some task. On a recent bike trip with a psychiatrist, he confided in me that his only recurrent dream was where he was playing in his college band (which he had not done in about 25 years). In the dream, he was always unprepared and had not practiced. Interestingly, Freud had noted that this dream only occurs with tasks where we have been actually successful in waking life. It is possible that the examination dream is an ancient archetypal dream where we might be undertaking a life-threatening task, like an animal hunt. By having the fear of being unprepared, the dreamer awakens and is consciously reminded by the anxiety of the dream to bring along enough spears, to sharpen the spears, to remember the ropes, etc. The examination dream may reflect threat rehearsal or an unconscious priming mechanism that upon awakening insures the success of the task, as noted in Chapter 4.

The dream of appearing nude or inappropriately dressed, as I have already noted for other dreams, may also be overdetermined (have more than one cause). However, its evolutionary roots are relatively transparent. Once I did a 75-mile bike trip through a 9500 ft Colorado mountain pass. My friend Mike and I, as had become typical, seriously misjudged how long it would take us. As we climbed the pass with just 15 miles to our hotel, it started to get dark, and it gets cold in Colorado at night anytime of the year, but particularly when you are biking over a 9500 ft mountain pass. We put on what little extra clothes we had, not thinking we might get caught out in the dark. I was freezing; I began to shiver with the first sign of hypothermia. There were no cars passing us. If we had stopped, we would have probably fallen unconscious and died from the cold. We had no choice but to continue shivering and pedaling. When we reached the summit, we had only five miles of coasting downhill to go. I remember my brief joy when we started to coast but a new fear struck! The wind-chill temperature! As we started to hit 30 miles an hour, I started to feel, in terror, numbness in my hands and feet. When we arrived at the hotel, I have never felt so good taking a hot shower. Thus, it is easy for me to imagine, especially when our ancestors were not so protected from their environment that their dreams of being nude or inappropriately dressed may have also served an unconscious priming function that later warns the conscious self of the Boy Scout motto: be prepared!

Finally, I have already discussed my first empirical study (Coolidge and Bracken, 1984) of the loss of teeth in dreams in Chapter 9. In the Jewish Talmud, the loss of teeth dream is interpreted as the future death of a family member. Even 4000 years ago, Egyptians interpreted the tooth-loss dream as the death of the dreamer by the machinations of one's relatives. Much later, Freud commented on the dream's association with death, and the Native American Navajo also thought it portended death of a family member. It is relatively easy to see how the dream might become associated with ancient ancestral fears of aging and death, because tooth loss later in the adult lifespan is concomitant with dietary changes and other physical changes that herald the end of our lives. Also, the loss of teeth may have been concomitant with muscular and strength changes that signaled a loss of power and physical prowess.

However, it is also important to remember that we do not lose our teeth for the first time in later adult life. Freud may have been right when he wrote that many dreams replay early childhood impressions. The tooth-loss dream may replay the losing of our baby teeth when we were young, and those early fears about losing our teeth may be retriggered in later adulthood, well before the actual physical loss of teeth. Thus, the tooth-loss dream may be relatively unique in that it may replay not only our phylogeny but also our ontogeny.

Jung

Jung attached far more significance to recurrent dreams than Freud. Jung even proposed three possibilities for recurring dreams:

> A dream of this kind is usually an attempt to compensate for a particular defect in the dreamer's attitude to life; or it may date from a traumatic moment that has left behind some specific prejudice. It may also sometimes anticipate a future event of importance.
> (Jung, 1968; p. 40)

Jung gave the example of his own recurring dream: he dreamt that he had discovered some new part of his house that he had not known existed before. He wrote:

> Sometimes it was the quarters where my long-dead parents lived, in which my father, to my surprise, had a laboratory where he studied the comparative anatomy of fish, and my mother ran a hotel for ghostly visitors. Usually this unfamiliar guest wing was an ancient historical building, long forgotten, yet my inherited property. It contained interesting antique furniture, and toward the end of this series of dreams I discovered an old library whose books were unknown to me. Finally in the last dream, I opened one of the books and found in it a profusion of the most marvelous symbolic pictures. When I awoke, my heart was palpitating with excitement.
> (Jung, 1968; p. 40)

Jung wrote:

> ...[T]he motif of my recurring dream can be easily understood. The house, of course, was a symbol of my personality and its conscious field of interests; and the unknown annex represented the anticipation of a new field of interest and research of which my conscious mind was at that time unaware. From that moment, 30 years ago, I never had the dream again.
> (Jung, 1968; p. 40)

I find it interesting that Jung thought it so easy to interpret his own recurring dream. He obviously thought the dream had only one meaning, his third type of recurring dream, the anticipation of some future event. I think it gives us some insight into the difficulties of interpreting our own dreams. First, Jung overlooked Freud's idea that the dream was a wish-fulfilling dream, and I can see at least two wishes in the dream: his long-dead parents are alive, and he finds some 'marvelous symbolic pictures' in a book.

Second, given that Jung claimed our shadow contains everything that we fear to acknowledge about ourselves, why could he not at least postulate that there may have been other possibilities for interpretation? Was Jung that consciously well defended? I think that he was and that helps clarify some of the trouble between Freud and Jung. Freud may have acted too paternally, autocratically, and dogmatically with Jung, but Jung had his own strong ego defenses. Freud claimed that Jung wished him dead. Jung always denied it, yet he had a dream about the time of their fateful breakup where Jung helped kill a man named Siegfried.

In defense of Jung and his interpretation of his own dream, Jung thought his own insight into his *own* dream was sufficient. Jung thought that dreams were not a facade, a dream's picture contains its entire meaning. There is no deception in dreams. Jung wrote:

> My intuition consisted of the sudden and most unexpected insight into the fact that my dream meant *myself*, *my* life and *my* world, my whole reality against a theoretical structure erected by another, strange mind for reasons and purposes of its own. It was not Freud's dream, it was mine; and I understood suddenly in a flash what my dream meant.
> (Jung, 1968; p. 44)

Two paragraphs later he wrote this strong affirmation of his dream position:

> The individual is the only reality. The further we move away from the individual toward abstract ideas about *Homo Sapiens*, the more likely we are to fall into error.
> (Jung, 1968; p. 45)

Also to Jung's credit, when he had finished interpreting his recurring house dream to his own immediate satisfaction, he said that he never dreamt about it again. This, of course, does not mean that Jung is correct in his assertions about recurring dreams, but it does mean that he obviously believed his assertions. Domhoff (1996) noted that clinical lore, based on studies and surveys, asserts that once the underlying problem has been solved, the recurrent dream will disappear.

Perls

Perls thought that the most important dreams were the recurring type. Perls objected to the Freudian notion that these dreams represented a kind of compulsive repetition leading to psychological petrification and death. Perls believed that the opposite was actually true. Perls thought that these dreams had the potential to help us solve major unfinished issues in our lives. Perls said:

> If something comes up again and again, it means that a gestalt has not been closed. There is a problem which has not been completed and finished and therefore can't recede into the background. So if anything, it's an attempt to become alive, to come to grips with things. And very often these repetitive dreams are nightmares. Again, it's the opposite from Freud who thought that dreams are wishful thinking. In the nightmares you find always how you frustrate yourself.
> (Perls, 1969a; p. 16)

Perls makes a salient point about nightmares as a type of recurrent dream. Again, as I mentioned earlier, empirical research more often than not has defined recurrent dreams vaguely. The themes in nightmares are often repeated, as Perls has noted, yet are rarely discussed as a specific type of recurrent dream, when they so obviously are. In the 1980s there were a number (Hartmann, 1984; Kramer, Schoen, and Kinney, 1987) of empirical investigations of the recurrent traumatic dreams of Vietnam veterans. This research has shown that the soldiers who were most likely to suffer from these dreams after their traumatic experiences were younger, less educated, and emotionally closer to someone who was killed or injured. Also, traumatic recurrent dreams appeared to dissipate and change into ordinary dreams over time, and did so more quickly with group therapy. A spontaneous recurrence of the traumatic dreams was also observed when new stressors like divorce entered the picture.

Summary

1 It appears that what constitutes a recurrent dream is vaguely defined throughout the literature.
2 Freud dismissed recurring dreams as simple childhood remembrances, and said he had never had one himself, but proceeded to give many examples of repeated people and themes from his dreams.
3 Jung thought recurrent dreams were important and gave three common types: a perceived defect in the dreamer, a trauma, or a future anticipation.
4 Perls also thought recurrent dreams were important, if not the most important type of dream, because Perls believed that recurrent dreams were attempts to solve major unfinished issues.
5 Current clinical lore suggests that recurrent dreams will dissipate with time or therapy, or if a solution to the underlying issue is discovered.

CHAPTER 11

A synthesis of dream interpretation techniques

In this final chapter I shall summarize some of the dream techniques that I have found most useful in interpreting dreams. I will also give numerous examples of my dream interpretation experiences from the classroom, dream workshops (e.g. Coolidge, 1999), and from therapy sessions.

> Principle 1: Dreams form a hierarchy of unfinished business.

Perls suggested that our psychological issues formed a hierarchy of unfinished business. Because I believe, like Freud, Jung, and Perls, that dreams contain elements of our past, present, and future, I think dreams have the potential to reveal deep secrets, repressed thoughts and problems, and issues on the edges of consciousness. I suggest listening very carefully to a person's dream. I strongly suggest not asking too many informational or logical questions about the individual's dream story. Take the dream at face value. However, I do recommend actively forming hypotheses about what unfinished business the dream story could contain. Your goal should be to bring forth some unfinished business to consciousness. As Freud said, where id was, ego shall be. Awareness, per se, is thought to be curative. From Perls' perspective, you should help dreamers become aware and re-own fragmented parts of their personalities.

Dream example 1: Duke, the neglected dog

A divorced woman in her forties shared this recurring dream: 'I had a Rottweiler named Duke and about five years ago I had to give him away because we were moving. He went to a very good home but I felt bad about it. About a year ago I started having this dream, which I've since had about five times. In the dream, I've forgotten I've had him [forgotten I still own him]. It dawned on me that I haven't fed him or watered him for weeks...'

At that very point I interrupted her. To me, the neglected dog was too compelling.

'Become Duke,' I said. She paused and looked at me, then away.

'Duke would say...' she started to say, and I interrupted again.

'No, no,' I said. 'You become Duke.'

'I love you anyway,' she said in a flat, monotone voice.

'Say it with more meaning,' I said.

'Without crying?' she asked, and she turned her head away with tears welling up in her eyes.

'Why did you cry?' I asked. 'What did that make you think about?'

As she regained her composure, she said, 'I grew up in a very legalistic family.'

I thought the choice of the word 'legalistic' was very intriguing, and I asked her about it. She said she was raised by her stepfather who she said was 'very unforgiving' and conditional. When I probed her about the latter description she said that he set up conditions which she felt obliged to follow, such as maintaining a weight he set for her, all A grades at school, etc. She said it was 'hell' living with him. And then she very quickly freely associated to what she described as another 'hellish' situation with her former husband who cheated on her.

At this point, she made the connection that saying 'I love you anyway' when she became Duke might be a message from her unconscious self to her conscious self. She pondered, without any additional questions or comments from me, whether she had truly begun to forgive herself for feeling so bad about her stepfather's unloving harshness and her ex-husband's cheating ways.

> Principle 2: People have a tendency to avoid and alienate the holes in their personalities despite their compensating need for wholeness. Watch for these holes in dreams.

Perls also pointed out that this tendency to dissociate and disown even occurs physically. Rather than saying, 'I am fingers,' we say, 'I have fingers.' It may also be considered a western phenomenon to locate the center of consciousness in our heads, which no doubt contributes to our dissociative tendencies. Easterners, particularly the Chinese and Japanese, are much more likely to ascribe the center of consciousness near the navel. In fact, one of the reasons that Buddha statues have big bellies is not only the connotation of health and wellbeing but also because Buddha possesses a belly-centered consciousness. One time on a river trip with my brother, I stood relaxed and contemplative on the banks of an oak tree-lined river, meditating on its pristine beauty. My brother came up and poked my belly and said unpoetically, 'You're getting a gut.' I countered, 'Ah, it is not a gut. I have belly-centered consciousness.'

Another sign of this dissociative process occurs when we say, 'I have a backache.' I once did a clinical internship in a campus counseling center. A fellow I saw for the first time said that he had been sent over from the medical center because:

'I have headaches.'

'When did they send you over,' I asked.

'A year ago,' he replied.

Immediately, I thought this fellow was guarded, distrusting of therapy and ambivalent. These hypotheses were also supported by his body language and general demeanor. The situation required some risky measures. I trusted that on some intuitive level, if I could show him some value of therapy, he might return. After all, although he took a year to get here, he was here. I decided to take the risk. The next thing I said to him was:

'Say: I am a headache.'

He said, 'What?' with some degree of skepticism.

I said, 'You told me you have headaches. I said tell it to me this way: I am a headache, instead of saying: I have a headache.'

He paused, looked at me, and said meekly, 'I am a headache.'

I said, 'Say it again but louder.'

I was getting anxious. I could feel it building. Would this work? Yet he said it again, and so I pressed him once more to say it like he really meant it.

Finally he said forcefully, 'I AM A HEADACHE. I AM A HEADACHE.' And then he added softly and sadly, 'I am a headache to myself.'

'How?' I asked. And therapy proceeded semi-smoothly for a full college quarter as we discussed his various self-defeating behaviors.

I had used Perls' techniques for making the patient take responsibility for dissociation and making the patient amplify a statement forcefully and meaningfully. I was also amazed that I had taken such risks in therapy, following my readings of Perls but also following my intuition. Moreover, we had arrived at a major unfinished issue for this fellow without a review of his family history, or even his dreams! Thus, we return to my original thesis statement and add to it.

We have a psychological tendency to complete tasks. Anxiety arises when we fail to complete them. As Perls noted we operate on a continuum of awareness, and the most important unfinished business eventually emerges into awareness. Perls also thought that we had hundreds of these unfinished issues that arrange themselves hierarchically. So we have a number one piece of unfinished business, a number two, etc. I point out to my classes that, no doubt, some issues sometimes take over number one but on a temporary basis: for example, when we worry about paying a certain bill, or studying for a test, etc. However, these issues come and go relatively quickly. I think Perls was referring to issues that would average number one over a long period of time. When I am listening to people's dreams, I have noticed that some issues tend to be in most people's hierarchy. For example, issues about death are common, not feeling the love of a parent, independence–dependence issues, etc.

Perls uses dreams to bring out the unfinished business. He achieves this by listening carefully to not only what the patient says, but also how they say it, their body language, and the melody of their entire demeanor. He said:

So how do we proceed in Gestalt Therapy? We have a very simple means to get the patient to find out what his own missing potential is. Namely, the patient uses me, the therapist, as a projection screen, and he expects of me exactly what he can't mobilize in himself. And in this process, we make the peculiar discovery that no one of us is complete, that every one has holes in his personality.

Now these missing holes are always visible. They are always there in the patient's projection onto the therapist... Then the therapist must provide the opportunity, the situation in which the person can grow. And the means is that we frustrate the patient in such a way that he is forced to develop his own potential. We apply enough skillful frustration so that the patient is forced to find his own way, discover his own possibilities, his own potential, and discover that what he expects from the therapist, he can do just as well himself.

So what we are trying to do in therapy is step-by-step to *re-own* the disowned parts of the personality until the person becomes strong enough to facilitate his own growth, to learn to understand where are the holes, what are the symptoms of the holes. And the symptoms of the holes are always indicated by one word; *avoidance*.
(Perls, 1969a; p. 36–8)

Now we have come to a major irony. Like Perls I do believe that dreams reveal our major unfinished businesses. However, in the strictest sense, *I do not interpret dreams and neither did Perls!* He wrote:

...we don't interpret dreams. We do something much more interesting with them. Instead of analyzing and further cutting up the dream, we want to bring it to life... Instead of telling the dream as if it were a story in the past, act it out in the present, so that it becomes a part of yourself, so that you are really involved.

If you understand what you can do with dreams, you can do a tremendous lot for yourself on your own. Just take any old dream or dream fragment, it doesn't matter. As long as a dream is remembered, it is still alive and available, and it still contains an unfinished, unassimilated situation. When we are working on dreams, we usually take only a small little bit from the dream, because you can get so much from even a little bit.
(Perls, 1969a; p. 68–9)

So the irony is that dreams are simply a vehicle to get at unfinished business. I do not care about the logic of the dream. I do not care to hear about endless dream characters, and story shifts. People are frequently disappointed when I do not let them finish telling me their long and boring dreams. I stop them as soon as I hear (and intuit) some interesting, provocative, compelling, or curious feature in the dream. At that point, I have the person become that object or person. Most of the time, I favor inanimate objects over people because most dreamers write scripts for the people in their dreams all too easily. Perls urged his dreamers to:

> ...write a script...ham it up. Really *become* that thing – whatever it is in a dream – *become* it. Use your magic. Turn into that ugly frog or whatever is there – the dead thing, the live thing, the demon – and stop thinking. Lose your mind and come to your senses. Every little bit is a piece of the jigsaw puzzle, which together will make up a much larger whole – a much stronger, happier, more completely *real* personality.
> (Perls, 1969a; p. 69)

Jung, even earlier than Perls, wrote about this dissociative process, the usefulness of dreams in reclaiming the unconscious, and the wholeness that results:

> In this respect, dream symbols are the essential message carriers from the instinctive to the rational parts of the human mind, and their interpretation enriches the poverty of consciousness so that it learns to understand again the forgotten language of the instincts.
> (Jung, 1968; p. 52)

Principle 3: Have the dreamer become part of the dream and write a script. I favor inanimate objects over animate objects in the dream.

When I have chosen the object I want the dreamer to become, I say to them: 'Become that object. What would it say if it could talk to you?' Sometimes, at this point, people stare at me incredulously. 'What do you mean?' they ask.

'Become the object,' I repeat. 'Pretend you are an actor or actress. Make it talk. Make it say something to you.'

Here I sometimes get from the dreamer, 'It would say...'And I stop them immediately. 'No. Become the object. Don't talk in the third person. Start with, 'I am... I feel...'

I would estimate that about 90% of the time, the dreamer will successfully generate some statement. Typically it is very short, maybe five to seven words. I have had two recent dreamers produce two words and three words respectively. Yet in both cases, the dreamers and I were satisfied that we had indeed discovered major unfinished issues.

Dream example 2: Take us out

The three-word example came from a 21-year-old former GI who was returning to college. He came to my office after a general psychology lecture. He said that

I had mentioned in class the dream about loss of teeth. He said that this dream was a recurrent one for him for the past four years. I asked him to describe the dream, and he said he had it at least once a week. He said that he usually wipes his mouth with the back of his wrist, and groups of his teeth, likes twos and threes will be on his wrist amidst blood.

'Become the teeth,' I said. 'What would they say to you?'

'Become the teeth?' he asked politely.

I nodded.

'Take us out,' he said. I was fascinated.

Principle 4: Listen carefully to the language of the dreamer.

I caution you, at this point, because I had a traumatic experience with a girl in the eighth grade over what she supposedly had said. I paraphrased what I thought she said to someone else. That someone told her what I said she had said. She found me in the hallway and gave me a tongue-lashing I have not forgotten. Suffice to say, do not attempt to paraphrase. Simply memorize, as best you can, by repeating out loud whatever the person says. In this case, I repeated, 'Take us out?' and he nodded.

Before proceeding any farther, however, I follow Perls' example of trying to enliven the statement, trying to make the dreamer own it, or trying to make the dreamer show some emotional involvement. So I said:

'Say it again but louder.'

'Take us out,' he said, virtually repeating the monotone way he first had said it.

'Say it again but mean it!' I said forcefully.

'TAKE US OUT,' he said loudly but still flatly, but I decided I had done enough skillful frustration for the present. I did not wish to ruin the rapport.

I said, 'What does that make you think about in your life?'

He paused reflectively. I kept myself stifled, enduring the pregnant silence.

'Nothing,' he said. I waited another slow pregnant moment.

I broke the silence but I recommend that you wait as long as necessary for the dreamer to say something first. I said:

'Who might you say that to in your life? Take us out!'

'No one,' he said softly after another long wait.

I think a bad hypothesis is better than no hypothesis so I said:

'Do you have a sibling?' I thought, perhaps, because the teeth in his dream were in twos and threes, that perhaps they symbolized siblings.

'Yes, a brother,' he said.

'Would you say that to your parents?' Here, I was thinking that maybe he and his brother were too sheltered, and he wanted his parents to take them to the movies, on vacation, etc.

'No,' he said animatedly. 'I love my parents.'

I suddenly realized I had misunderstood his phrase. To him, 'Take us out,' meant something bad. So I asked him. Indeed, he said it meant to get rid of something, like wipe it out.

'Let's take it as a message to yourself,' I said. 'Make your teeth, in groups of twos and threes, talk to you and say, 'Take us out!' What might that mean to you?'

He paused again. 'I think I know,' he said.

'What?' I asked gently.

'There's parts of me I don't like. I'd like to get rid of some things.'

'Like what?' I said.

'I'm an introvert. I wish I could just change that. Take it out.'

'Well, I think that's one of the meanings of your dream,' I said.

Next, I tested whether he thought that this issue was an important one for him (high in his hierarchy). He agreed without hesitation.

It is important to point out a difference between Freud and Perls on this point. If a dreamer said no to this question, in other words, saying that this was not a very important issue for them, Perls would accept it. Perhaps, the therapist was simply wrong, Perls reasoned. It is possible, of course, despite our good intuitions and our best hypotheses. Freud would probably have taken the 'no' as a sign of unconscious resistance (or even of denial and conscious resistance) to the truth of the hypothesis. What if you still feel your interpretation is correct but the person is denying it? Perls said it is possible that you are right but it is not yet time for the dreamer to admit it. Be patient.

> Principle 5: Everything in the dream is a projected aspect of the dreamer. However, unfinished psychological issues can be raised by having a person create a script with anything. This technique can be used with people who say they do not dream.

Virtually everyone dreams. People who swear that they do not dream come into the sleep lab, have electrodes attached to their heads, go to sleep, go into REM sleep, and then they are awakened. Invariably they smile. I tried this twice in graduate school with friends. Why do they smile? Because they were dreaming, and they swore to me they did not, yet I got them to admit they were dreaming vividly.

So the issue appears to be that some people do not remember their dreams. The solution is simple. Simply becoming aware about dreams seems to help people to remember. When I worked in the sleep lab, I would go home, and I would have dreams I was working in the sleep lab and monitoring people's sleep on the EEG. Some people find that if you put a pad of paper and a pencil beside your bed before you go to sleep, it seems to help the memory for dreams. Also, encourage those who say they do not remember their dreams to write down their dreams before getting out of bed. It is well known that dreams are forgotten quickly upon awakening. If you are sleeping with another person and you both awaken at the same time, telling each other your dreams is another good mnemonic technique.

Dream example 3: Gone fishing

A woman about 35 years old was in my Principles of Counseling class at the university. We covered a section on dream interpretation in psychotherapy. She told me she never remembered a dream.

'Never?' I asked.

'Never,' she said firmly.

'Not a bit, not a fragment, not a childhood dream, a nightmare, nothing?' I asked incredulously.

'Nothing,' she said in what seemed like a sinister way.

'Well,' I said cockily. 'Put some paper and a pencil beside your bed before you go to sleep. When you awaken try to remember something about your dreams. Anything. And do not go to the bathroom first. The dream will fade quickly if you do.'

We met five days a week. So the next day, I looked forward to my success. Everyone was given the homework to bring in a dream – recent, recurring, a nightmare, or any remembered dream fragment. As soon as we assembled, I looked right at her.

'So?' I said.

'Nothing,' she smiled.

'Did you put a pencil and paper beside your bed?' I asked.

'No,' she said, 'because I knew it wouldn't work.'

I made a face of incredulity. The class giggled.

'Humor me,' I said, pretending to be weak with frustration. 'Try it!' I added.

The next day in class, she came in with a sheepish look.

'I don't believe it,' she said. 'I don't remember dreaming, but when I woke up I found that some time during the night I had written this, and she handed me a sheet of paper with two words on it: 'Gone fishing.' The class eagerly awaited my interpretation.

'I think this could be a message to yourself,' I said. 'What does it make you think about?'

'I don't know,' she said appearing truly perplexed.

'Think about your unfinished business,' I said (we had already covered Perls and Gestalt Therapy so she was familiar with the language). 'What could the message mean?' I added.

She paused and pondered and then she lit up like a light bulb.

'Oh, I know,' she said. 'I need a vacation.'

I remained quiet. Something was welling up inside her. Her voice became more confident.

'I am a single mother with three kids. I'm trying to go through this masters program. I get no help whatsoever from my ex, his parents, or my parents. I have to be the responsible one for everything, every minute of the day and night. Just once, I'd like to put up a sign that says, 'Gone fishing.'

'Do you think that this is an issue for you that you'd benefit by sharing in therapy?' I asked.

'Of course,' she said. 'It's my biggest issue.'

Note that I try to assess how well I have hit the person's hierarchy of unfinished business. I have given examples where I have succeeded. On occasion, I do miss. Either the dreamer tells me it is an issue but they do not feel it a very important one, or they tell me they do not feel it is an issue at all. The latter circumstance is rare, however. It simply is not hard to generate some topic for therapy with this dream technique.

Most of the time, the technique works so easily that I am reminded of Jung's warning:

> This episode [a colleague's free association] opened my eyes to the fact that it was not necessary to use a dream as the point of departure for the process of 'free association' if one wished to discover the complexes of a patient. It showed me that one can reach the center directly from any point of the compass. One could begin from Cyrillic letters, from meditations upon a crystal ball, a prayer wheel, or a modern painting or even casual conversation about some trivial event. The dream was no more and no less useful in this respect than any other starting point. Nevertheless, dreams have a particular significance, even though they often arise from an emotional upset in which the habitual complexes are also involved. [The habitual complexes are the tender spots of the psyche, which react most quickly to an external stimulus or disturbance.] That is why free association can lead one from any dream to the critical secret thoughts.
>
> At this point...it might reasonably follow that dreams have some special and more significant function of their own... I therefore began to consider whether one should pay more attention to the actual form and content of a dream, rather than allowing 'free association' to lead one off through a train of ideas to complexes that could easily be reached by other means.
> (Jung, 1968; p. 27–8)

I would argue with Jung on three counts. First, I admit that the dream techniques I am using appear to involve free association. However, it is not clear to me that the material I end up discussing with the dreamer could have been reached by any other means. Second, with very few exceptions, I am always using the dream to direct my inquiry. I am not using a crystal ball. I am using a dream. Jung himself proposed that the dreams should direct therapy. The techniques I am using do just that. Third, even if all that I am reaching are 'habitual complexes,' I do not feel that is a simple feat. Patients enter therapy with conscious and unconscious resistances and lifetimes of dissociations and alienation. If, in the space of only five minutes, my patient and I are discussing something that, by their own admission, is an important topic (high in their hierarchy of unfinished business) who am I or who is Jung to disagree!

In fact, Jung himself said that dream symbols are, by definition, hidden, vague, and ultimately unknowable. I think one could err, much more readily, in the opposite direction, by wasting the patient's time turning a dream over and over again. Jung even stated that dreams should be accepted as facts, and dreams are specific expressions of the unconscious. If a woman tells me that her dream told her to go fishing, then I am not about to argue with her or the wisdom of her dream interpretation. In fact, delaying that message would be absurd.

Dream example 4: No dream, no time

In dream seminars where I lecture for a single session, if someone says that they do not dream, I do not have the luxury of sending them home to sleep beside a pencil and paper. This is where I make my single exception to trying to reach the hierarchy of unfinished business by way of a dream. In a general psychology class, for example, a woman about 25 years old, who had raised her hand, said she never remembered a dream or even a fragment.

I said, 'Imagine when you wake up and there's this dream that you don't remember in your room. What would that dream say to you as you are lying in bed.'

'Why don't you remember me?' she said.

'What would you say back to the dream?' I asked.

'You're not important. You don't matter,' she said with a sudden kind of sad realization in her voice.

'You thought of something in your hierarchy?' I asked gently.

'Yes,' she said, and I pressed no further. I thanked her for being so brave in front of the class.

Dream example 5: Don't eat here!

In another recent dream seminar, in front of community college students, I asked the class for a recurring dream. The first person to volunteer was a 28-year-old woman who said she dreamt repeatedly of a hostage situation at a fast food restaurant. She told me the dream that simply and quickly. I was forced to think quickly and thought she could either become a hostage or the restaurant. Because I always prefer inanimate objects, I told her to become the restaurant.

'You want me to become the restaurant?' she asked with doubt.

'Yes. Just like an actress. Become the restaurant. What would you say?'

'I'd say, don't eat here.'

The class laughed.

Because I had already given the class at least a one-hour or more introduction to sleep, dreams, and Perls' idea about unfinished business in dreams, I asked them to generate possibilities for unfinished business in her statement.

'She doesn't like fast food,' said someone.

'She doesn't like restaurants,' said another.

I was disappointed because I felt these suggestions were simply manifest meanings. 'No,' I said, 'think big unfinished issues. Life issues.'

A man about 40 years old sitting in the back raised his hand and said, 'Maybe she doesn't like living here. Maybe food is like a connection to a place. Like sustenance. Maybe she'd like to move and eat. I mean like live somewhere else.'

'OK,' I said. 'That's better. Don't just sit there. Think. A bad idea is better than no idea. Are there any other ideas?'

'Stop,' said the woman with the dream. 'That's it,' she said, shaking her head with firm resignation. 'I don't want to live here,' she added. But before she could continue, I thanked her for sharing with us.

Dream example 6: Don't take me

A 40-year-old female acquaintance recently approached me with a dream. She was currently going through a divorce and had two young children.

'I dreamt that my husband came to my house with a pick-up truck, and he was towing a cement mixer, and three large big things,' she said.

'Become the three large big things,' I said, because I'm attracted to inanimate objects in dreams and the bizarre. 'What would they say?' I said.

'Like what?' she said.

Listening and remembering carefully to exactly how she phrased it, I repeated, 'What would the three large big things say if they could speak?' I said.

She paused. When people pause anything over about three seconds, I remind them not to think too hard. I encourage them to say just what first comes up. She had paused more than three seconds, so I said, 'Don't think too much. What would they say?'

'Don't take me,' she said with life and meaning behind it so I did not ask her to repeat it. She said it with real feeling.

'What does that make you think about in your life?' I asked.

'Oh, my kids. They hate going with their father. And I feel so guilty.'

'In what way?' I asked.

'Oh, they don't want to go with him. At the same time, it's not just that they'd rather stay with me. They'd rather have us get back together but that's just not gonna happen. I can't tell them that.'

'Well, that's what I think one of your dream meanings might be,' I said.

'What about the feeling I had in the dream that after he visits me with these vehicles, he's gonna leave my house empty? I think it means I feel like he's cleaning me out,' she added somewhat questioningly.

I affirmed the meaning she gave to her dream without hesitation, agreeing with Jung that it is her dream, her life, her interpretation. However, I did feel that she might ultimately benefit by becoming conscious of how her children's fantasies about reconciliation were on a collision course with her future plans.

Dream example 7: Move me

A 27-year-old female, newly married, undergraduate came to my office for a dream interpretation session. She said she started college at 17 years old, had attended three different colleges, and was now in her tenth year of college studies. She said in her dream she was in an old house in a bad part of town with lots of old cars strewn about. She said her niece was in front of the house, and the niece was excited because Sam (the co-ed's ex-husband) was coming to visit. Next, she said, a large man came up and was collecting money. She said that she told him they (she and her niece) did not have any money. Behind the house, she said she then spied a kitten sitting really still.

At that point, I said, 'Become the kitten. What would the kitten say to you?'

'Move me, get me out of here,' she said, and giggled.

I said, 'What does that make you think about? You giggled.'

She said without hesitation, 'My family. They drive me crazy.'

I immediately thought about Hartmann's theory that dreams contextualize emotions. In this dream, I thought about her car metaphor (old cars strewn about) and even the subtle statement of, 'they *drive* me crazy.' But my intuition told me that this was perhaps the manifest meaning of the dream, in part because her association between the kitten and her family came so easily. So I returned to her original dream statement.

'Say what the kitten said again,' I said.

She said, 'Move me and get me out of here.'

I said, 'What does that make you think about in your present life?'

She paused and said, 'I don't know.' She then paused again looking thoughtful. After a pause of about 20 to 30 seconds, she said, 'I hold myself back.'

'How?' I asked.

'In so many ways,' she said. 'I make all kinds of excuses so I won't meet new people. I keep myself full of anxiety. I make things up to block myself from doing new things. I really believe in spirits and possibilities but I hold myself back.'

She paused again and then said, 'I've been thinking about this for a while. I use to blame my parents for delaying me in school and holding me back but I realize I am the one holding myself back.'

I then told her that dreams probably have many meanings but that I found it meaningful that after only about five minutes in my office, we were talking about her holding herself back. I told her I just could not believe that was random or by accident. I told her that she probably had just been given a letter from herself to herself (like the sixteenth-century dream interpreter Almori) and that she was now fulfilling her responsibility (like the twenty-first century sleep expert

Hartmann) by examining the meanings of her dream. I also told her that it is common for psychologists to believe that awareness, per se, may be curative, and I also explained that her awareness of these issues would undoubtedly help her in her journey to finish school and stop holding herself back from new people and things that she wanted to do.

Dream example 8: Stuck in time and place

Liz [not her real name] is a 21-year-old daughter of one of my neighbor's friends. She had heard about my dream work and wanted to try it out. We sat outside on my front porch and she began right away without any prompting.

'This dream is really long so cut me off,' she said. 'I start by going to a large building. I run into a tour guide, an older man, and he introduces himself as my tour guide. First, we go into a room with one giant fan and several smaller fans in the walls. All of the fans are frozen with ice on them.'

I stopped her

'Become the frozen fans. What would they say to you?'

'Stuck in time or place,' she said, with little hesitation

'What does that phrase mean to you?' I asked.

'I'm not moving,' she said.

'What do you mean?' I asked.

'I feel like I've already spent too much time in school. I've changed majors three times. I wish I could go back in time five years. I could even deal with my family better.'

I said, 'How?'

'I've got nine siblings. There have always been these alliances between the siblings. It's like we need to form alliances to defend ourselves from the other siblings and from our parents. But I never did. I'm on the outside. So they call me asking me to fix things for them and to help them. But they are all stubborn. They all live in the past. They are all stuck in their ways. I'm the only one in school right now. My issue with all of them is their rigidity. But it worries me, and I keep things in. I don't make other people help me like they do. I think I should be able to fix my own problems. But I'm perfectionistic too so I have a lot to live up to.'

She kept on talking freely. I nodded and gave her nonverbal support. After a few minutes, she seemed to wind down. I reinforced her search for her own identity outside of being one of ten children. And I told her a bit of my dream ideas. I also told her that at 21 years old, she actually had not spent that much time in school and to go easier on herself in that regard. She left rather happily.

Dream example 9: Some dreams are wish-fulfilling

One of my research assistants came to me with a dream she wanted interpreted. She is 25 years old and engaged to be married. She said she dreamt that her fiancé's mother was sick and died from cancer. She said in reality she's 'healthy as a horse.'

This seemed like a classic mother-in-law issue, so I raised the possibility with her that the dream might conceal a hidden wish, but this is how I deflected resistance at the outset:

'Freud said *all* dreams are wish-fulfilling but I don't believe that. But I do believe some dreams are wish-fulfilling, and I have a feeling this might be one of them. Is there some way you would like to be rid of your future mother-in-law?' I said.

'I really like her. She talks a ton but she's generous, loving, and has a great heart,' she said.

'How might it be nice to be rid of her?' I asked again.

'I guess I'd like to show his side of the family that I can be strong like her. I can plan things just like her. She's a wedding planner...' she said, as I interrupted.

'As a profession?' I asked.

'Yes, she's a professional wedding planner, and she's planned this huge reception for our wedding, and I don't want a huge reception. She's also planned a huge wedding, which we don't really want but we'll do it for her, but we don't want both a huge wedding and huge reception. Yet she keeps telling me it's my day, it's my day.'

'And then you dream that she dies,' I said. 'Why are dreams so mysterious?' I asked facetiously, and we both laughed.

As I review my own techniques, I think back to what Carl Jung said about dream interpretation. Learn as much as you can about dream interpretation and then forget it. I know that I eclectically choose among the various ideas of Freud, Jung, Perls, and others. I choose what seems to fit the occasion. I rely heavily on my intuition. I try to remember that there's no single hidden meaning every time. I won't always be successful. I won't always have a very satisfied person leave my office. But I do recognize that it's fairly easy to hit some issue or unfinished business in a dream. And very often, I do have people leave my office who believe that I have raised a singularly important piece of unfinished business. I usually reinforce the notion that awareness, per se, is curative, and advise them to seek professional help if they ever feel overwhelmed, and I tell them I can refer them to someone really good if they feel they ever need it.

In this dream, my intuition immediately suggested the classic Freudian wish-fulfilling dream notion, and it appeared to work. She was able to voice some conscious concerns that she said she had shared with no one other than her future husband. I also told her that, by voicing those concerns through her dreams and by sharing them, she had not actually settled her issues with her future mother-in-law but she was on the road to settling them. I told her I believed that she was now, at least theoretically, less likely to have an accident involving her mother-in-law where her mother-in-law would be hurt. Again, we laughed.

Dream example 10: I can help

A man in his early thirties shared this dream in one of my dream workshops. He first told us that he had trained as a nurse in the army and had returned to college to get his prerequisites for dental school. He then told us that this dream recurred with great regularity when he was younger (less than 15 years old) but that he occasionally still had it. In his dream, he was on Gilligan's Island with the regular cast. He said Santa Claus' sleigh with Santa's toy bag inside would suddenly land in the midst of the group. He said that was essentially the whole dream.

'Become Santa's toy bag,' I said.

'I can help,' he said rather quietly and because of, in part, the ambient noise of the large group, and also my feeling that he was reluctant to say it loudly, I said:

'Louder!'

He said, 'I CAN HELP!'

I said, 'How does that fit your life?'

Without pausing, he almost sheepishly said: 'It's my life's theme.'

'How?' I asked.

Without hesitation, he related that since very early on in his family, he took on the role of a helper. He then made it his profession, first becoming a medical technician and then joining the army and becoming a nurse. He then said it was a role that he did not always cherish.

'Can you think of ways it has been both a blessing and a curse?' I asked.

He said, 'Easily.'

And I suggested to the participants of the dream workshop that this is where therapy might begin, that is, it begins with his recognition that helping others has been both beneficial to him but that it appears he now has some idea that the role might have also been at some psychological cost.

Principle 6: Listen carefully and be patient.

A dear colleague of mine, and friend for over two decades, said he would write a quote for the cover of my dream book. It would say: 'This is a good book but the techniques only work for Fred.' As many times as he has seen me use the technique successfully, he says he fails miserably. I've heard him try it a couple of times in my presence. I think he does not pause long enough after he asks them to think about what their dream script statement makes them think of in their lives. If you knew this wonderful fellow, you would see the irony, because he is famous for his long and thoughtful pauses. So I encourage you to be patient.

Aristotle reflected, nearly 2400 years ago, on what it takes to be an interpreter of dreams. He wrote:

The most skillful interpreter of dreams is he who has the faculty of observing resemblances. Anyone may interpret dreams which are vivid and plain. But speaking of 'resemblances,' I mean that dream presentations are analogous to the forms reflected in water, as indeed we have already stated. In the latter case, if the motion in the water be great, the reflexion has no semblance to its original nor do the forms resemble the real objects. Skillful indeed, would he be in interpreting such reflexions who could rapidly discern, and at a glance comprehend, the scattered and distorted fragments of such forms, so as to perceive that one of them represents a man, or a horse, or anything whatever. Accordingly, in the other case also, in a similar way, some such thing as this [blurred image] is all that a dream amounts to; for the internal movement effaces the clearness of the dream.
(Aristotle, 1952c; p. 709)

I think that the skillful interpreter of dreams is one who listens carefully and is patient. I think there is a wonderful metaphor for dream interpretation in the book *Siddhartha* by Hermann Hesse (1951) (which Perls also mentions in *Gestalt Therapy Verbatim*). Vasudeva, the ferryman, tells the hero of the story, Siddhartha, to listen to the river (which may be a metaphor for a dream):

'You will learn it,' said Vasudeva, 'but not from me. The river has taught me to listen; you will learn from it, too. The river knows everything; one can learn everything from it. You have already learned from the river that it is good to strive downwards, to sink, to seek the depths. The rich and distinguished Siddhartha will become a rower; Siddhartha the learned Brahmin will become a ferryman. You have also learned this from the river. You will learn the other thing, too.'

After a long pause, Siddhartha said: 'What other thing, Vasudeva?'

Vasudeva rose. 'It has grown late,' he said, 'let us go to bed. I cannot tell you what the other thing is, my friend. You will find out, perhaps you already know. I am not a learned man; I do not know how to talk or think. I only know how to listen and be devout; otherwise I have learned nothing. If I could talk and teach, I would perhaps be a teacher, but as it is I am only a ferryman and it is my task to take people across this river. I have taken thousands of people across and to all of them my river has been nothing but a hindrance on their journey...however, amongst the thousands there have been a few, four or five, to whom the river was not an obstacle. They have heard its voice and listened to it, and the river has become holy to them, as it has to me. Let us now go to bed, Siddhartha.'
(Hesse, 1951; p. 68)

In summary, I suggest that you try to feel comfortable with even a small success. Do not worry too much about trying to solve all of other people's major unfinished issues. Try, instead, to help the dreamer understand a small part. As Perls wrote:

> And if you understand the meaning of each time you identify with some bit of the dream, each time you translate an *it* into an *I*, you increase in vitality and in your potential...you get, let's say, a ten-thousandth of your potential back, and it will accumulate. Each time you can integrate something it gives you a better platform, where again you can facilitate your development, your integration.
> (Perls, 1969a; p. 71)

Summary

1 Dreams form a hierarchy of unfinished business.
2 People have a tendency to avoid and alienate the holes in their person-alities despite their compensating need for wholeness. Watch for these holes in dreams.
3 Have the dreamer become part of the dream and write a script. I favor inanimate objects over animate objects in the dream.
4 Listen carefully to the language of the dreamer.
5 Everything in the dream is a projected aspect of the dreamer. However, unfinished psychological issues can be raised by having a person create a script with anything. This technique can also be used with people who say they do not dream.
6 Listen carefully and be patient.

References

Aeschylus (1935) Agamemnon. In: J Gassner *A Treasury of the Theatre*. Simon and Schuster: New York, NY.

Allison T and Cicchetti DV (1976) Sleep in mammals: ecological and constitutional correlates. *Science*. **194**: 732–4.

Almori (1848) – as incorrectly cited by Freud. See Covitz (1990) for a translation of Almori's original 1515 work.

American Psychiatric Association (2000) *Diagnostic and Statistical Manual of Mental Disorders* (DSM-IV-TR). American Psychiatric Association: Washington, DC.

Aristotle (1952a) On sleep and sleeplessness. In: MJ Adler (ed) *Great Books of the Western World*. Brittanica: Chicago, IL.

Aristotle (1952b) On dreams. In: MJ Adler (ed) *Great Books of the Western World*. Brittanica: Chicago, IL.

Aristotle (1952c) On prophesying by dreams. In: MJ Adler (ed) *Great Books of the Western World*. Brittanica: Chicago, IL.

Artemidorus (1975) *The Interpretation of Dreams: Oneirocritica* (RJ White, trans). Noyes Press: Park Ridge, NJ.

Aserinsky E and Kleitman N (1953) Regularly appearing periods of eye motility and concomitant phenomena. *Science*. **118**: 273–4.

Aubrey JB, Smith CT, Tweed S *et al.* (1999) Cognitive and motor procedural tasks are dissociated in REM and stage two sleep. *Sleep Research Online*. **2**: 220.

Barrett D (1996) *Trauma and Dreams*. Harvard University Press: Cambridge, Massachusetts.

Beatty J (1995) *Principles of Behavioral Neuroscience*. Brown & Benchmark: Dubuque, IA.

Bently P (1995) *The Dictionary of World Myth*. Duncan Baird Publishers: New York, NY.

Berger H (1930) Uber das elektrencephalogram des Menschen. *Journal of Psychiatry and Neurology*. **40**: 160–79.

Blagrove M (1992) Dreams as the reflection of our waking concerns and abilities: A critique of the problem-solving paradigm in dream research. *Dreaming*. **2**: 205–20.

Breasted JH (1912) *A History of Egypt*. Charles Scribner's Sons: New York, NY.

Brautigan R (1968) *In Watermelon Sugar*. Dell Publishing Co., Inc.: New York.

Budge EA (1978) *An Egyptian Hieroglyphic Dictionary: Vol. 1*. Dover: New York, NY.

Cartwright R and Lamberg L (1992) *Crisis Dreaming: using your dreams to solve your problems*. HarperCollins: New York.

Coolidge FL (1974) Memory consolidation as a function of sleep and the circadian rhythm. (Doctoral dissertation, University of Florida, 1974) *Dissertation Abstracts International*. **36B**: 0934.

Coolidge FL (1999, August) *Dream Interpretation as a Psychotherapeutic Technique*. Continuing Education Workshop presented at the annual meeting of the American Psychological Association, Boston, MA.

Coolidge FL and Bracken DD (1984) The loss of teeth in dreams: an empirical investigation. *Psychological Reports.* **54**: 931–5.

Coolidge FL and Fish CE (1983) Dreams of the dying. *Omega.* **14**: 1–8.

Coolidge FL and Salk P (in press) The meaning of teeth loss dreams in college students: a failure to replicate. Manuscript submitted for publication.

Coolidge FL, Thede LL and Young SE (2002) The heritability of gender identity disorder in a child and adolescent twin sample. *Behavior Genetics.* **32**: 251–7.

Coolidge FL and Wynn T (in press) *The Evolution of Modern Thinking.* Blackwell: New York.

Covitz J (1990) *Visions of the Night: a study of Jewish dream interpretation.* Shambhala Publications, Inc: Boston, MA.

Dawood NJ (1956) *The Koran.* Penguin: New York, NY.

de Becker R (1968) *The Understanding of Dreams and their Influence on the History of Man.* Hawthorn Books, New York, NY.

Dement W (1972) *Some Must Watch While Some Must Sleep.* WH Freeman: San Francisco.

Dement WC and Vaughan C (1999) *The Promise of Sleep.* Delacorte Press: New York.

Domhoff GW (1996) *Finding Meaning in Dreams: a quantitative approach.* Plenum Press: New York.

Donn L (1988) *Freud and Jung.* Charles Scribner's Sons: New York, NY.

Fischer S, Hallschmid M, Elsner AL *et al.* (2002) Sleep forms memory for finger skills. *Proceedings of the National Academy of Sciences USA.* **99**: 11987–91.

Freud S (1920/1990) *Beyond the Pleasure Principle.* WW Norton & Company: New York.

Freud S (1900/1956) *The Interpretation of Dreams.* Avon: New York, NY.

Gais S, Plihal W, Wagner U and *et al.* (2000) Early sleep triggers memory for early visual discrimination skills. *Nature Neuroscience.* **3**: 1335–9.

Gay P (ed) (1989) *The Freud Reader.* WW Norton & Company, Inc: New York.

Geisel TJ (1962) *Dr. Seuss' Sleep Book.* Random House: New York, NY.

Gould S (1985) *The Flamingo's Smile: reflections in natural history.* WW Norton & Company: New York.

Gould S (1986) Evolution and the triumph of homology, or why history matters. *American Scientist.* **74**: 60–69.

Gregor T (1977) *The Mehinaku: the dream of daily life in a Brazilian Indian village.* University of Chicago Press: Chicago.

Hanh TN (1991) *Peace is Every Step.* Bantam: New York, NY.

Hartmann E (1967) *The Biology of Dreaming.* Charles C. Thomas: Springfield, IL.

Hartmann E (1984) *The Nightmare: the psychology and biology of terrifying dreams.* Basic Books: New York.

Hartmann E (1998) *Dreams and Nightmares: the new theory on the origin and meaning of dreams.* Plenum Press: New York, NY.

Hartmann E (2001) *Dreams and Nightmares: the origin and meaning of dreams.* Perseus: New York, NY.

Heatherton TF and Weinberger JL (eds) (1994) *Can Personality Change?* American Psychological Association: Washington, DC.

Hess WR (1954) *Diencephalon, Automatic and Extrapyramidal Functions.* Grune & Stratton: New York, NY.

Hesse H (1951) *Siddhartha.* New Directions Publishing Corp: New York, NY.

Hill CE (1996) *Working with Dreams in Psychotherapy.* The Guildford Press: New York.

Hobson JA (1988) *The Dreaming Brain.* Bantam Books: New York, NY.

Hobson JA (1994) *The Chemistry of Conscious States*. Little, Brown and Company: Boston, MA.

Hobson JA and McCarley RW (1977) The brain as a dream state generator: An activation-synthesis hypothesis of the dream process. *American Journal of Psychiatry*. **134**: 1335–48.

James W (1890/1981) *The Principles of Psychology*. Harvard University Press: Cambridge, MA.

Jouvet M (1980) Paradoxical sleep and the nature-nurture controversy. *Progress in Brain Research*. **53**: 331–46

Jouvet M (1999) *The Paradox of Sleep: the story of dreaming*. The Massachusetts Institute of Technology Press: Cambridge, MA.

Jung CG (1968) *Man and His Symbols*. Dell: New York, NY.

Jung CG (1969) *Flying Saucers: a modern myth of things seen in the skies*. New American Library: New York.

Jung CG (1970) *Psychological Reflections*. Princeton University Press: Princeton, NJ.

Karni A, Tanne D, Rubenstein BS, *et al.* (1994) Dependence on REM sleep of overnight improvement of a perceptual skill. *Science*. **265**: 679–82.

Kavanau JL (2002) REM and NREM sleep as natural accompaniments of the evolution of warm-bloodedness. *Neuroscience and Biobehavioral Reviews*. **26**: 889–906.

Kramer M, Schoen L and Kinney L (1987) Nightmares in Vietnam veterans. *Journal of the American Academy of Psychoanalysis*. **127**: 67–81.

Krippner S and Hughes W (1970) Genius at work. *Psychology Today*. **June**: 40–43.

LaBerge S (1985) *Lucid Dreaming*. Ballantine: New York.

Lennon J and McCartney P (1966) Extract from the lyrics to *I'm Only Sleeping*. Revolver Album.

Levy CM, Coolidge FL and Stabb LC (1972) Paired associate learning during EEG-defined sleep: A preliminary study. *Australian Journal of Psychology*. **24**: 219–25.

Loran S (1957) Dream interpretation in the Talmud. *International Journal of Psychoanalysis*. **38**: 92–7.

Maquet P, Schwartz S, Passingham R *et al.* (2003) Sleep-related consolidation of a visuomotor skill: Brain mechanisms as assessed by functional magnetic resonance imaging. *Journal of Neuroscience*. **23**: 1432–40.

Morrison AR (1983) Paradoxical sleep and alert wakefulness: variations on a theme. In: MM Chase and ED Weitzman (eds) *Sleep Disorders, Basic and Clinical Research*. Spectrum: New York.

Palmer M (1986) *T'ung Shu*. Shambhala: Boston.

Perls FS (1969a) *Gestalt Therapy Verbatim*. Real People Press: NY.

Perls FS (1969b) *In and Out the Garbage Pail*. Real People Press: Lafayette, California.

Pinel JPJ (1993) *Biopsychology*. Allyn & Bacon: Needham Heights, MA.

Ray JD (1976) *The Archive of Hor*. Egypt Exploration Society: London.

Reiser MF (1990) *Memory in Mind and Brain*. BasicBooks: New York, NY.

Revonsuo A (2000) The reinterpretation of dreams: An evolutionary hypothesis of the function of dreaming. *Behavioral and Brain Sciences*. **23**: 877–901.

Ribeiro S, Goyal V, Mello CV *et al.* (1999) Brain gene expression during REM sleep depends on prior waking experience. *Learning & Memory*. **6**: 500–508.

Robbins P and Houshi F (1983) Some observations on recurrent dreams. *Bulletin of the Menninger Clinic*. **47**: 262–5.

Sabater Pi J, Veá JJ and Serrallonga J (1997) Did the first hominids build nests? *Current Anthropology*. **38**: 914–16.

Sagan C (1977) *The Dragon of Eden*. Random House: New York, NY.

Shostak M (1981) *Nisa, the life and words of a !Kung woman*. Harvard University Press: Cambridge, MA.

Siegel JM (2001) The REM sleep-memory consolidation hypothesis. *Science*. **294**, 1058–63.

Smith C and MacNeill C (1994) Impaired motor memory for a pursuit rotor task following Stage 2 sleep loss in college students. *Journal of Sleep Research*. **3**: 206–13.

Stickgold R, James L and Hobson JA (2000) Visual discrimination learning requires sleep after training. *Nature Neuroscience*. **2**: 1237–8.

Toth LA and Verhulst SJ (2003) Strain differences in sleep patterns of healthy and influenza-infected inbred mice. *Behavior Genetics*. **33**: 325–36.

Turkheimer E (2000) Three laws of behavior genetics and what they mean. *Current Directions in Psychological Science*. **9**: 160–64.

Van de Castle RL (1983) Animal figures in fantasy and dreams. In: A Kacher and A Beck (eds) *New Perspectives on our Lives with Companion Animals*. University of Pennsylvania Press: Philadelphia.

Van de Castle RL (1994) *Our Dreaming Mind*. Ballantine: New York, NY.

Vertes RP and Eastman KE (2000) The case against memory consolidation in REM sleep. *Behavioral and Brain Sciences*. **23**: 867–76.

Von Franz M as cited in Jung C (1964) *Man and his Symbols*. Dell Publishing Co: New York.

Wagner U, Gais S, Haider H *et al.* (2004) Sleep inspires insight. *Nature*. **427**: 352–5.

Walker MP (2005) A refined model of sleep and the time course of memory formation. *Behavioral and Brain Sciences*. **28**: 51–104.

Walker M, Brakefield T, Morgan A *et al.* (2002) Practice with sleep makes perfect: sleep dependent motor skill learning. *Neuron*. **35**: 205–11.

Walker MP, Brakefield T, Seidman J *et al.* (2003) Sleep and the time course of motor skill learning. *Learning & Memory*. **4**: 275–84.

Watson JB (1919) *Psychology from the Standpoint of a Behaviorist*. JB Lippincott Company: Philadelphia, PA.

Webb WB (1975) *Sleep, the Gentle Tyrant*. Prentice-Hall: Englewood, Cliffs, NJ.

Wilson MA and McNaughton BL (1994) Reactivation of hippocampal memories during sleep. *Science*. **265**: 676–9.

Wing Y, Lee S and Chen C (1994) Sleep paralysis in Chinese: ghost oppression phenomenon in Hong Kong. *Sleep*. **17**: 609–13.

Winson J (1985) *Brain and Psyche: the biology of the unconscious*. Doubleday/Anchor Press: New York.

Winson J (1990) The meaning of dreams. *Scientific American*. **Nov**: 89–96.

Wundt W (1896) *Lectures on Human and Animal Psychology*. Swan Sonnenschein & Co: London.

Wynn T and McGrew WC (1989) An ape's view of the Oldowan. *Man*. **24**: 283–98.

Ying Xu, Padiath QS, Shapiro RE *et al.* (2005) Functional consequences of a CKId mutation causing familial advanced sleep phase syndrome. *Nature*. **434**: 640–44.

Index